A Colour Atlas of Rheumatology

Published by Wolfe Medical Publications Ltd, 1974
Printed by Graphos, Arte Sobre Papel, Barcelona, Spain
ISBN 0 7234 0753 3 Cased Edition
ISBN 0 7234 0960 9 Limp Edition
New and enlarged edition 1980
Reprinted 1986

This book is one of the titles in the series of Wolfe Medical Atlases, a series which brings together probably the world's largest systematic published collection of diagnostic colour photographs.
For a full list of Atlases in the series, plus forthcoming titles and details of our surgical dental and veterinary Atlases, please write to Wolfe Medical Publications Ltd, Wolfe House, 3 Conway Street, London W1P 6HE.

General Editor, Wolfe Medical Atlases:
G. Barry Carruthers, MD(Lond)

A Colour Atlas of
Rheumatology

A C Boyle

MD FRCP

formerly
Director
Department of Rheumatology
The Middlesex Hospital
London

Wolfe Medical Publications Ltd

Contents

Preface

This colour atlas is not intended as a textbook, nor does it claim to be a complete record of the many manifestations of the rheumatic diseases. It simply sets out to show by clinical pictures, radiographs and histological specimens some of the more common (and a few of the less common) conditions encountered in the field of rheumatology.

Rheumatology has been one of the fast expanding fields of medicine during the past ten years, and no attempt has been made to cover the therapeutics of the various diseases described, since rapid advances in this aspect of the subject would out-date the book before publication. In addition, it was felt impossible to include many of the troublesome soft tissue lesions which confront the Rheumatologist, since so few of these are amenable to illustration.

It is hoped that the book will be of help to the senior medical student or the busy family doctor, neither of whom will usually have the time to delve into large textbooks for help in the diagnosis of rheumatological problems.

I am grateful to many of my colleagues at the Middlesex Hospital who have helped by providing some of the illustrations, and to Dr Barbara Ansell for some of the illustrations of juvenile chronic arthritis. Finally, my thanks to my secretaries Juliet Shackel and Gabrielle Reilly for much work done out of hours with cheerful forbearance.

A.C.B.

Introduction

Rheumatology is the study of connective tissue diseases and the medical disorders of the locomotor system.

Because pain, swelling or stiffness of joints, or muscular pain with or without wasting may form part of the clinical picture of a wide spectrum of diseases, it is difficult to define its boundaries, and the Rheumatologist must be prepared for the fact that many patients suffering from diseases outside the range of his own special interest may present to him with a complaint of 'rheumatism'.

Many of the soft tissue lesions which come within the province of the Rheumatologist are of relatively small importance and are usually self-limiting, whereas affection of joints (arthritis) is a major cause of misery and crippledom in all populations.

Arthritis disables a very large number of patients, and by virtue of the fact that its course is usually protracted and progressive and that death from it is uncommon, it absorbs a substantial proportion of available medical care. In addition as a consequence of the disability it so often causes, it may present serious social and economic problems for the patient, and on a national scale is one of the major causes of absence from industry.

Numerically, degenerative joint disease is the greater problem, but in the main is much less disabling than the forms of inflammatory arthritis. Of the latter, rheumatoid arthritis is by far the most important disease because it is so common and so often progresses to the stage when the sufferer may eventually become partially or totally dependant upon others. The table overleaf lists some of the more common causes of arthritis, and in the text which follows are illustrated those which come within the particular province of the Rheumatologist.

Some of the more common causes of arthritis

Bacterial
Staphylococcus
Gonococcus
Tuberculosis
Brucellosis

Blood diseases
Leukaemia
Myelomatosis
Haemophilia
Sickle cell disease

Connective tissue diseases
Systemic lupus erythematosus
Polyarteritis nodosa
Polymyositis
Systemic sclerosis

Degenerative
Osteoarthrosis
Spondylosis

Endocrine
Acromegaly
Hyperparathyroidism
Myxoedema

Enteropathic
Ulcerative colitis
Regional ileitis
Viral hepatitis
Whipple's disease

Hypersensitivity states
Serum sickness
Drugs

Metabolic
Gout
Chondrocalcinosis
Haemochromatosis
Alkaptonuria

Neuropathic
Syphilis
Diabetes
Syringomyelia

Pulmonary
Hypertrophic pulmonary osteoarthropathy
Sarcoidosis

Unknown
Rheumatic fever
Rheumatoid arthritis
Reiter's syndrome
Psoriatic arthritis
Ankylosing spondylitis

Viral
Rubella
Glandular fever
Mumps
Measles

1 Rheumatoid arthritis

In spite of intensive research rheumatoid arthritis remains a disease of unknown origin. Although its most obvious manifestation is a sub-acute or chronic relapsing polyarthritis, it should be remembered that it often also gives rise to a severe disturbance of general health (malaise, anaemia, weight loss etc.), and may be complicated by involvement of most of the body systems. Attempts to prove an infective basis for it have so far failed, nor can it be said for certain that disturbances of immune mechanisms are either a cause or an effect of the disease.

The disease is common; figures given for most populations vary between 1.6–5%. Although it may occur at any age, there is a peak for both sexes in the early forties. Women are afflicted four times more commonly than men and in general have a poorer prognosis. Heredity appears to play little part in its aetiology although familial clustering is sometimes observed.

The tendency of some clinicians to prefer the name 'rheumatoid disease' draws attention to the widespread systemic manifestations which may accompany the polyarthritis, yet to the patient these are generally unimportant in the light of progressive disablement from painful, stiffened, and deformed joints.

The essential pathological changes within the joints can conveniently be divided into four stages:

Stage I This is basically a synovitis, the synovial membrane becoming hyperaemic and oedematous with foci of infiltrating small lymphocytes. Effusion into the joint cavity will show a high cell count (5 000–60 000 per mm^3), with a predominance of polymorphonuclear leucocytes. X-rays will as yet show no destructive changes, but soft tissue swelling or osteoporosis may be seen.

Stage II The inflamed synovial tissue now proliferates and begins to grow into the joint cavity across the articular cartilage, which it gradually destroys. X-rays will now show narrowing of the joint space due to loss of articular cartilage.

Stage III The pannus of synovium having destroyed the articular cartilage by now partially fills the joint cavity, and erosions begin to appear in sub-chondral bone. X-rays will show extensive cartilage loss, erosions around the margins of the joint, and deformities may have become apparent.

Stage IV In this final stage of the disease the inflammatory process will be subsiding, and fibrous or bony ankylosis of the joint will end its functional life.

Changes similar to those found in the joints may occur in tendon sheaths and bursae. Subcutaneous nodules are often the hall mark of severe disease and characteristically contain a central area of necrotic fibrous and granulomatous material surrounded by a palisade of connective tissue cells inside an outer zone of chronic inflammatory cells. Perivascular foci of small round cells may also be seen in striated muscle and in the endoneurium and perineurium of peripheral nerves.

The most serious lesions occur in the arterial tree, sometimes presenting as a non-necrotising arteritis of the small terminal arterioles, but occasionally taking the form of a fulminating arteritis with a close resemblance to polyarteritis nodosa, and with the prospect of a fatal outcome for the patient.

In its most typical form, rheumatoid arthritis runs a course of exacerbations and remissions with a gradual advance of destructive changes in the joints. Nevertheless, studies suggest that up to 40% of patients have the disease in a mild form, and that it is only 10% of those affected who eventually become totally disabled. The ultimate prognosis is notoriously unpredictable, but an insidious onset, high ESR or a high titre of rheumatoid factor, episcleritis or evidence of vasculitis are usually signs of serious import.

The illustrations which follow show some of the more important manifestations of the disease.

The joints

1 Early rheumatoid arthritis of the hands. Although sometimes starting as a monarthritis, this disease usually begins as a symmetrical polyarthritis, the finger joints commonly presenting the earliest manifestations of pain, swelling and stiffness most marked in the early morning. As seen here, spindle swelling of the proximal interphalangeal joints, and swelling of the 2nd and 3rd metacarpophalangeal joints are characteristic. The left wrist shows marked swelling over the ulnar styloid, and it is in this situation that the earliest erosive changes may be detected on X-ray. Flexor tendinitis in the palm of the hand is also an early clinical sign, and may be detected by palpating the flexor tendons in turn while the corresponding finger is passively flexed and extended.

2 In the early stages of rheumatoid arthritis X-rays may be entirely normal. In sequence are: (1) soft tissue swelling around affected joints with peri-articular osteoporosis; (2) joint space narrowing due to cartilage destruction; (3) rheumatoid erosions around joint margins. Note well-marked cartilage loss in the right 3rd metacarpophalangeal joint, and erosion of the right 2nd metacarpophalangeal joint. An early erosion is present at the distal end of the left 1st metacarpal bone, and overall there is juxta-articular osteoporosis.

1

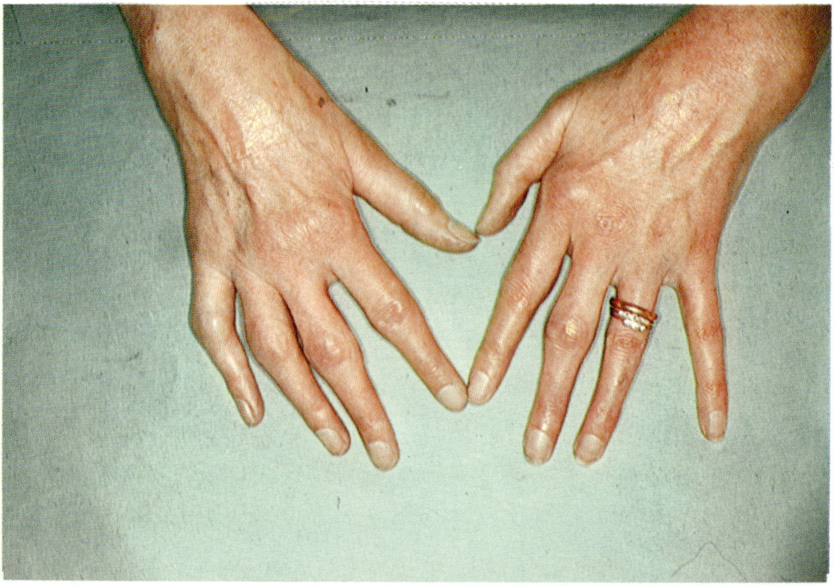

2

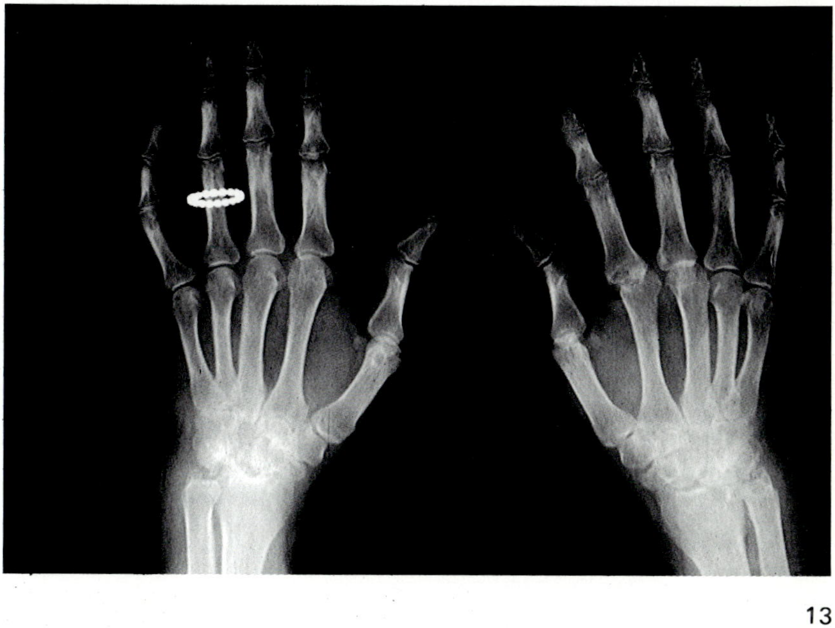

3 Proximal interphalangeal joint showing progression of rheumatoid changes from normality (on the left), to severe erosion (on the right). The interval between these films was 2 years.

4 Severe rheumatoid arthritis of the hands. Progressive and long-standing disease may result in deformity, subluxation, or ankylosis of the joints. Ulnar deviation of the fingers is typical of the later stage of the disease, and severe muscle wasting with large tendon sheath effusions may also be seen. Note the 'swan neck' deformity of the fingers shown in this figure together with massive tendon sheath swelling over the dorsal surfaces of both wrists and the severe muscle wasting.

3

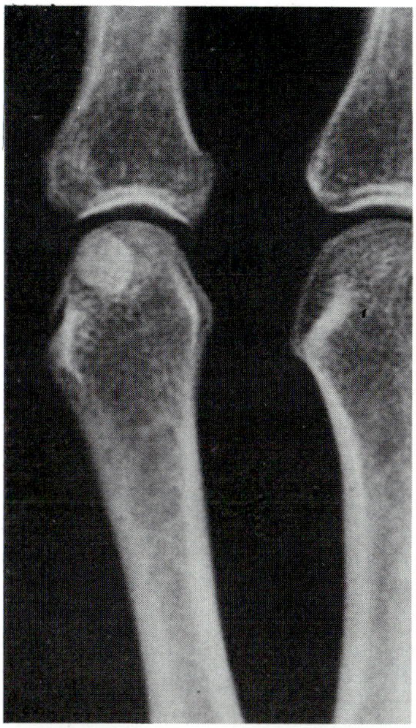

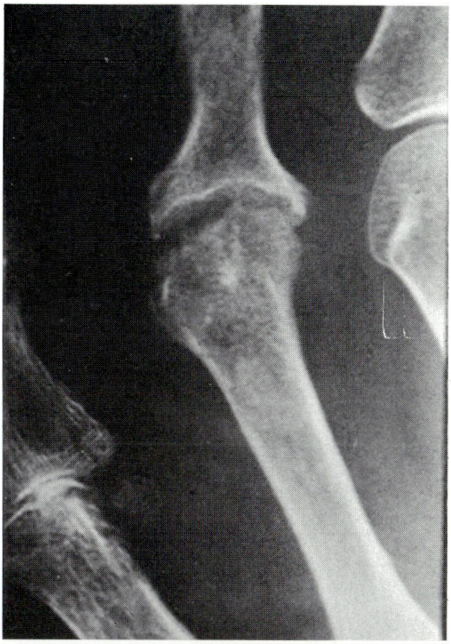

4

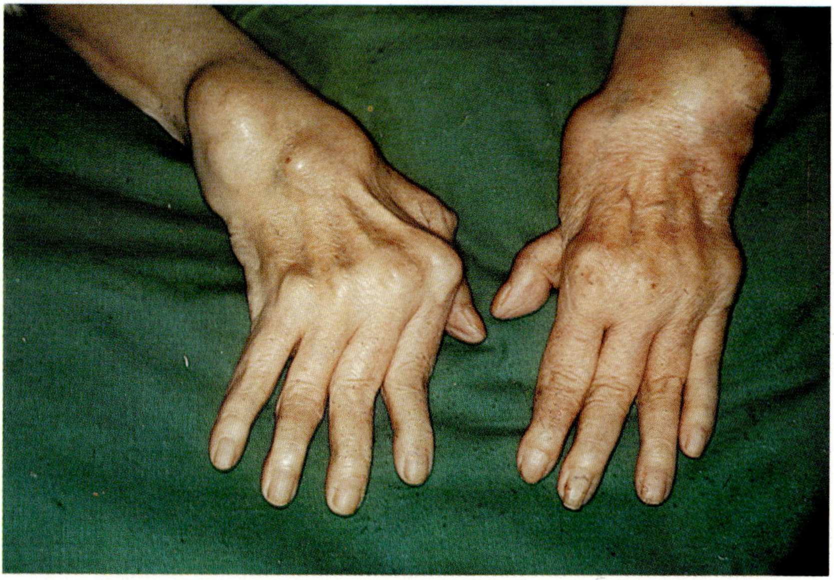

5 **Profound osteoporosis** with extensive destructive changes and subluxation of many of the finger joints.

6 **'Liver palms'** are associated with severe and longstanding disease.

7 **Tenderness and swelling of the metatarsophalangeal joints:** the feet are usually affected early. Fibular deviation of the toes may occur at a later stage.

5

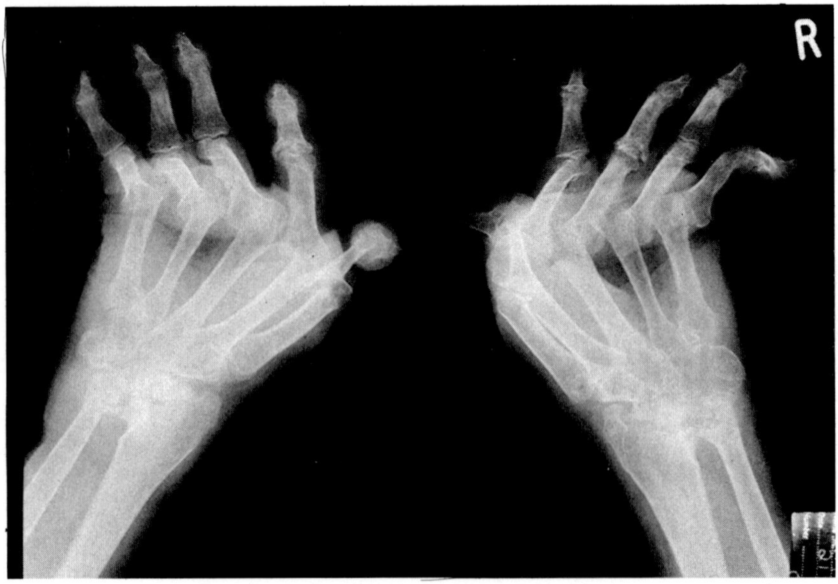

6

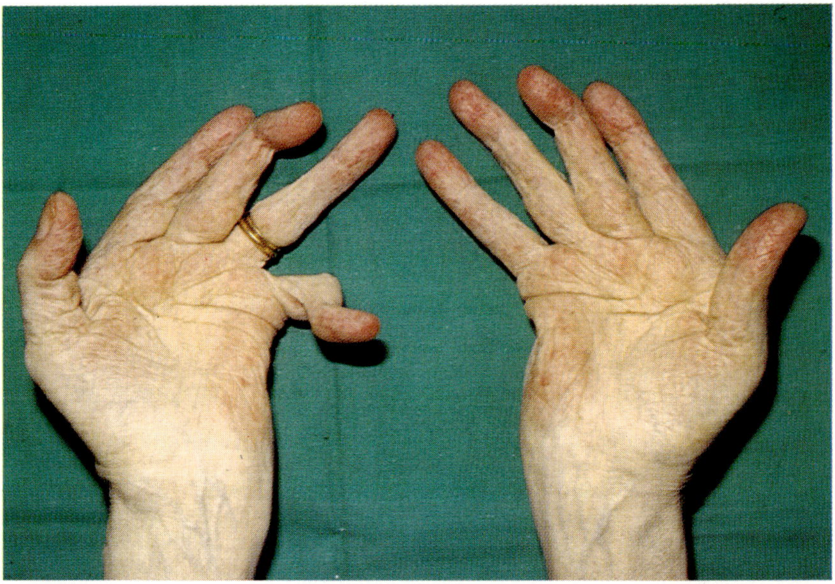

7

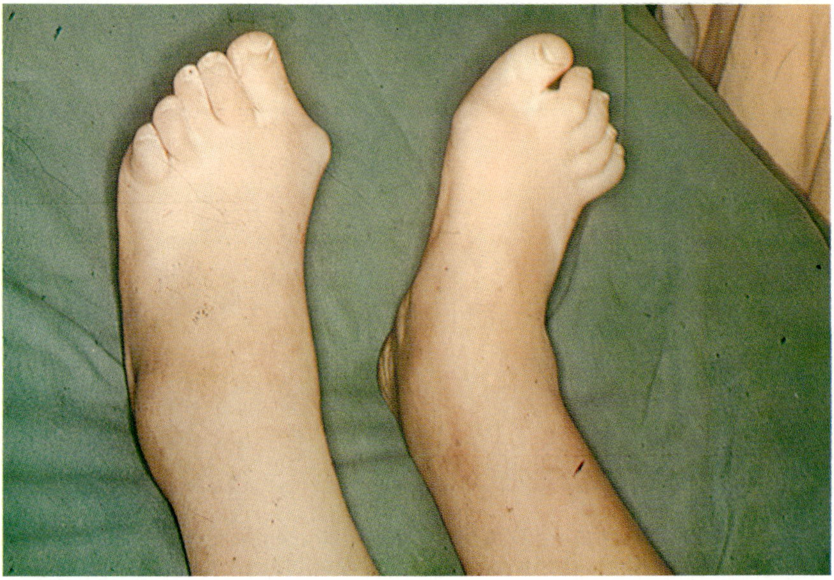

8

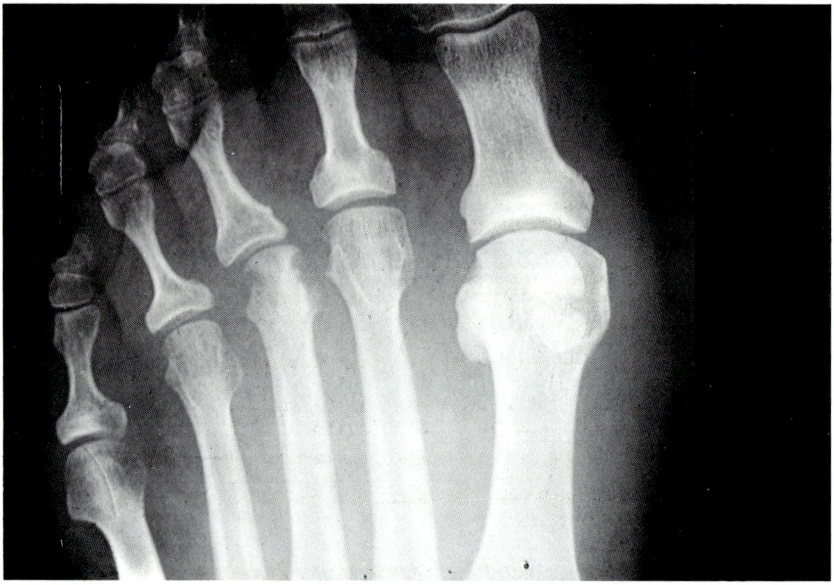

8 Cartilage loss and erosions affect the 3rd metatarsophalangeal joint. Radiological changes in the feet sometimes precede similar changes in the hand.

9

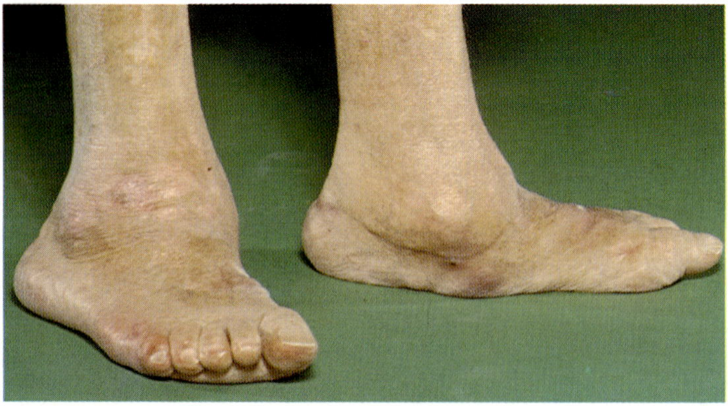

9 Advanced rheumatoid arthritis of the feet usually proceeds to collapse of the tarsus with resulting painful eversion deformity, as shown here.

10

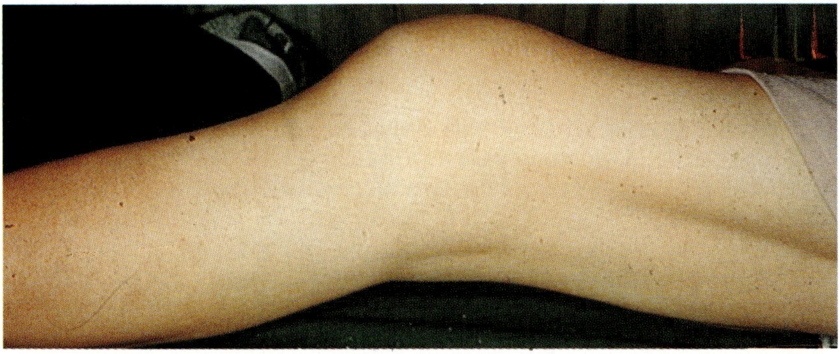

10 Knees are commonly involved, presenting with warmth and effusion within the joint. Flexion contracture is apt to occur early and should be carefully watched for. Continuing inflammation may later involve the lateral and cruciate ligaments leading to instability.

11 Early rheumatoid arthritis of the knee showing loss of joint space and an early erosion of the lateral tibial plateau (*arrowed*).

11

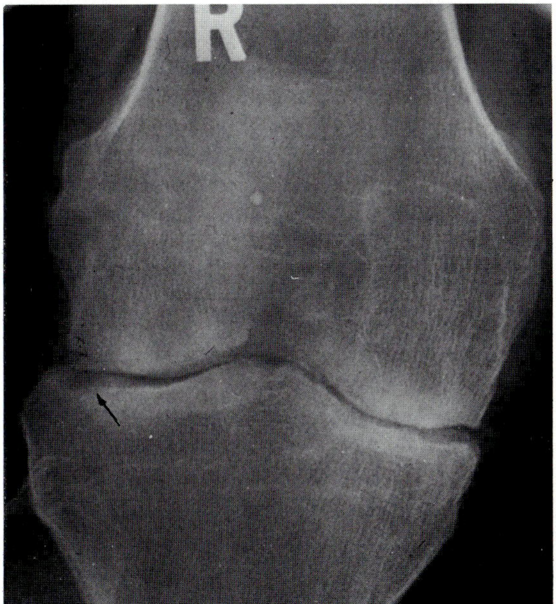

12 Advanced rheumatoid arthritis of the knee. Note almost total cartilage loss and erosion of the medial tibial plateau and medial femoral condyle.

13 Weight bearing on an eroded and osteoporotic knee may sometimes lead to collapse of the tibial plateau as seen here on the lateral side of the joint. The patient may complain of sudden exacerbation of pain following undue activity.

14 Rupture of the synovial membrane of the knee is not uncommon, when the effusion tracks down into the calf muscles. The patient presents with an acute painful swelling in the posterior aspect of the calf. Differential diagnosis from a deep vein thrombosis may present a problem.

15 Advanced rheumatoid changes in both knees with valgus deformity of the right knee. Swelling of the left calf is due to a synovial rupture.

16 Posterior view of the same patient (**15**).

12

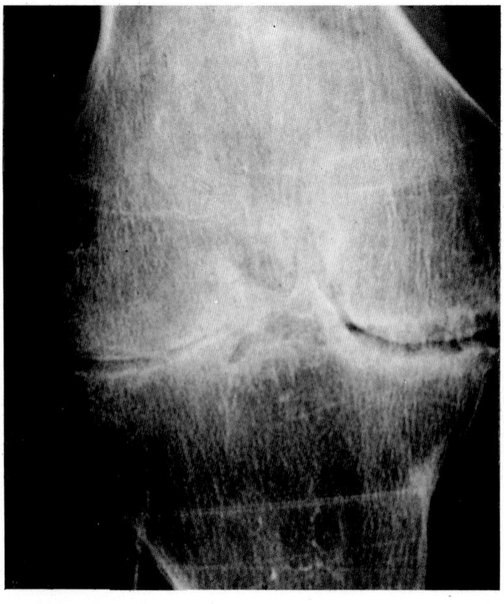

13

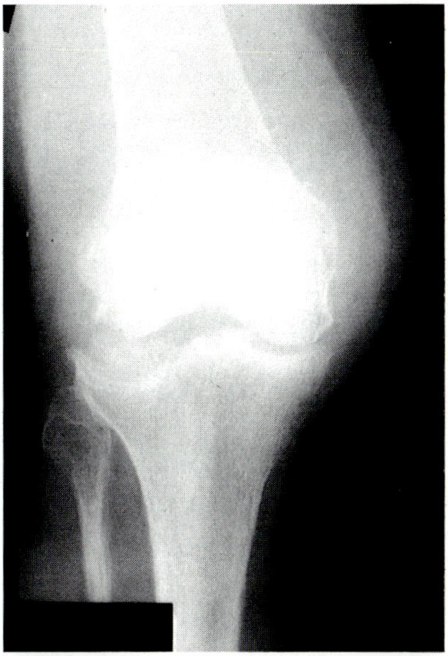

14

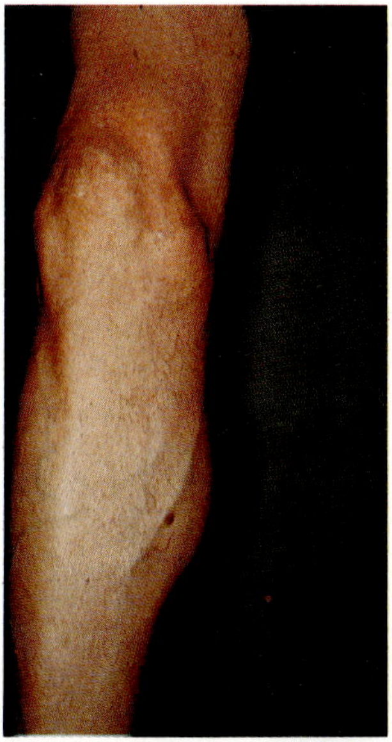

15

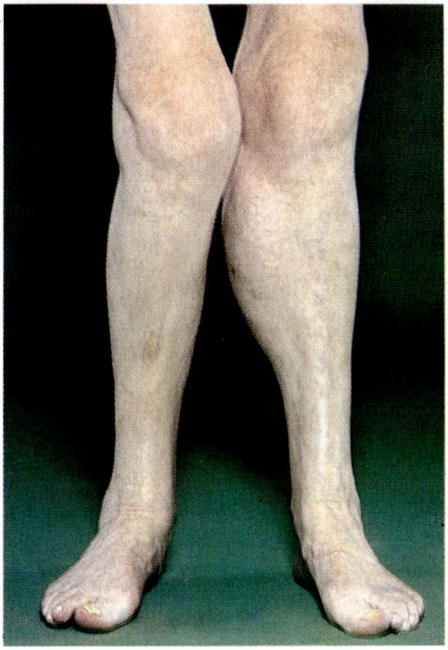

16

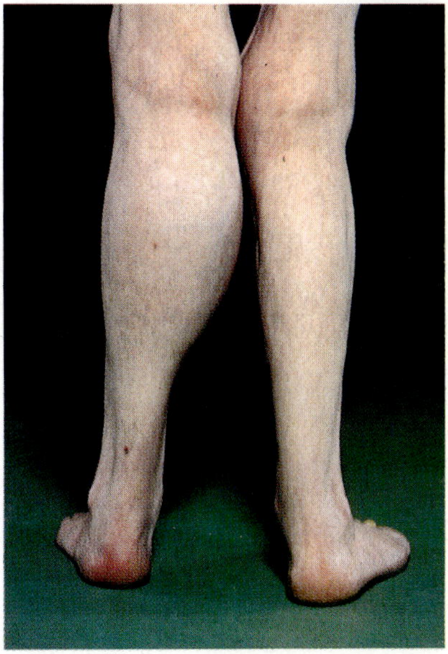

17 Ruptured knee joint. Arthrogram showing the dye tracking down into the calf.

18 Early rheumatoid arthritis involving right hip joint. There is cartilage loss and erosion of the femoral head and of the roof of the acetabulum. Involvement of the hip usually causes severe pain which may be resistant to medical treatment.

19 Moderate rheumatoid arthritis of the hip joint. There is even cartilage loss and extensive erosions of the femoral head.

17

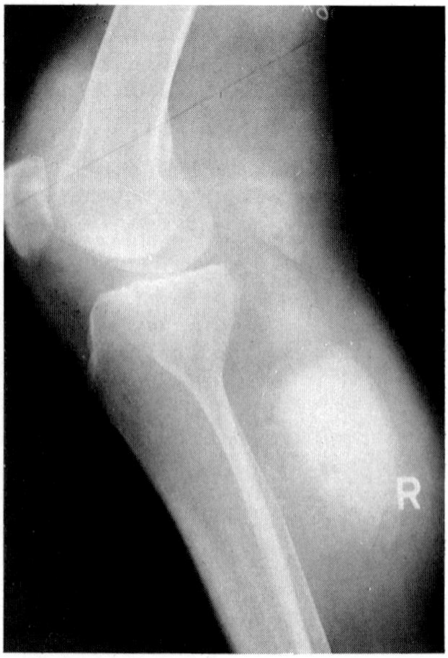

18

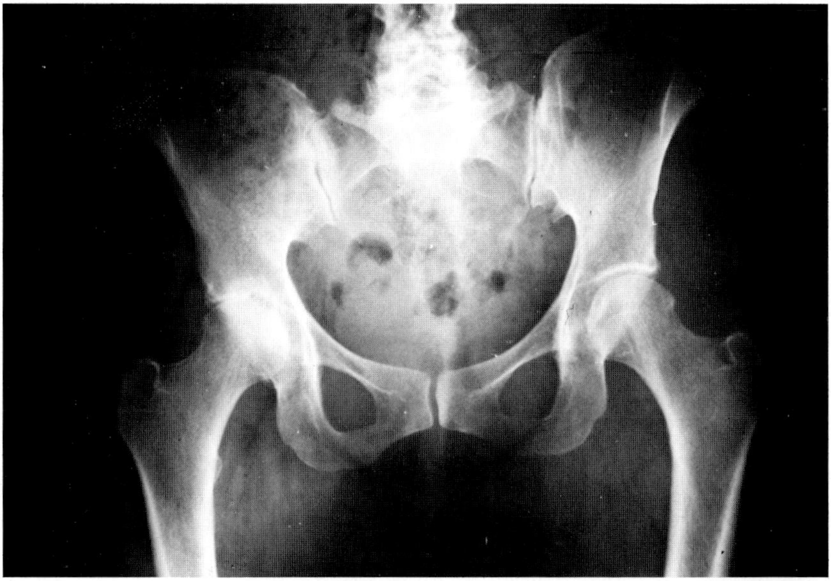

19

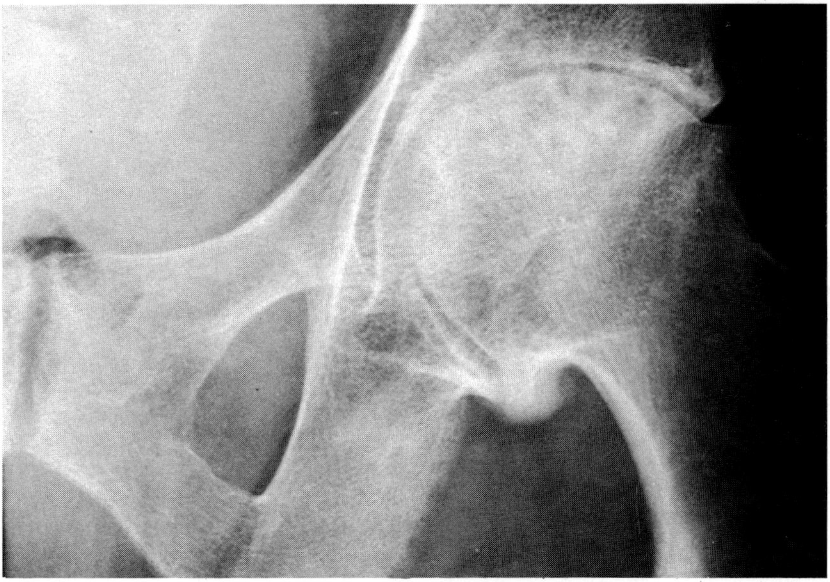

20 Advanced rheumatoid arthritis of the hips. As with other types of inflammatory arthritis protrusio acetabuli may occur as shown in this X-ray.

21 Rheumatoid arthritis of the shoulder joint. If effusion occurs it usually presents anteriorly. Even in early involvement of the shoulder severe restriction of movement may be present before radiological changes are seen.

22 Advanced rheumatoid arthritis of the shoulder. Note destructive changes involving the humeral head, with upward dislocation. The acromioclavicular joint is also severely eroded.

20

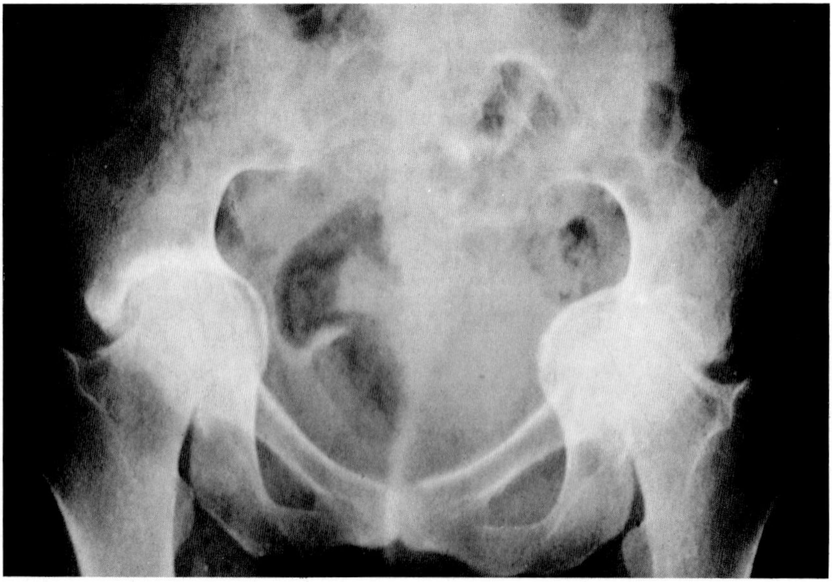

21

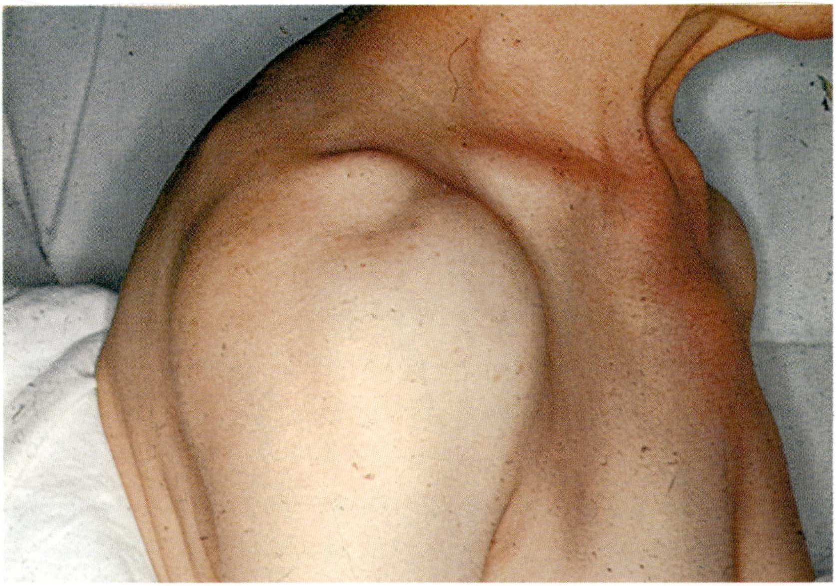

22

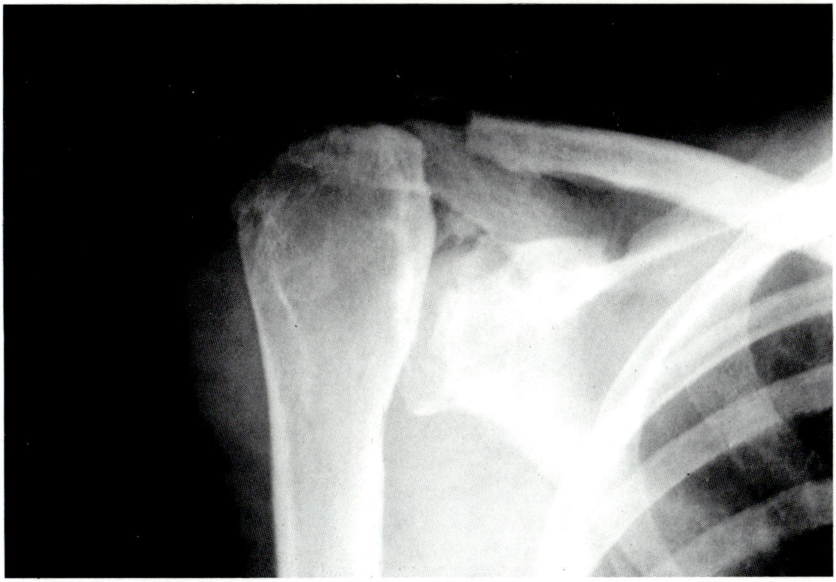

23

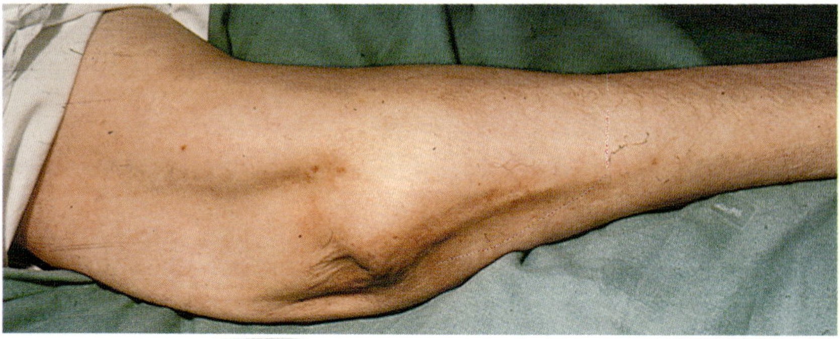

23 Involvement of elbow often causes considerable disability and restriction of movement. Limitation of extension precedes loss of other movements. Compression of the ulnar nerve may occur (see page 54).

24 Advanced involvement of elbow. Note almost complete destruction of cartilage and erosion of the radial head and lateral humeral epicondyle. Large rheumatoid cysts are more commonly seen in the elbow than any other joint.

24

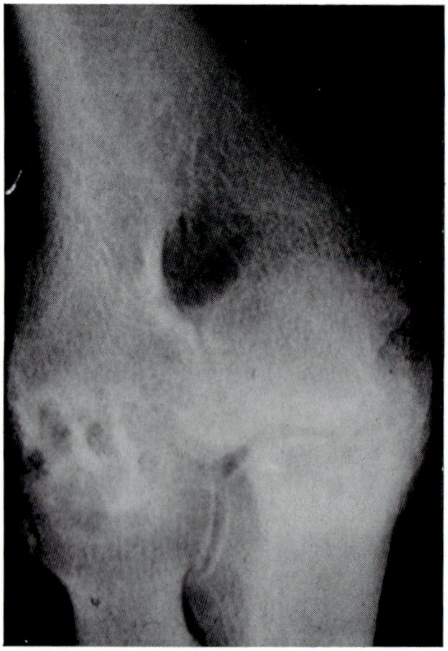

25

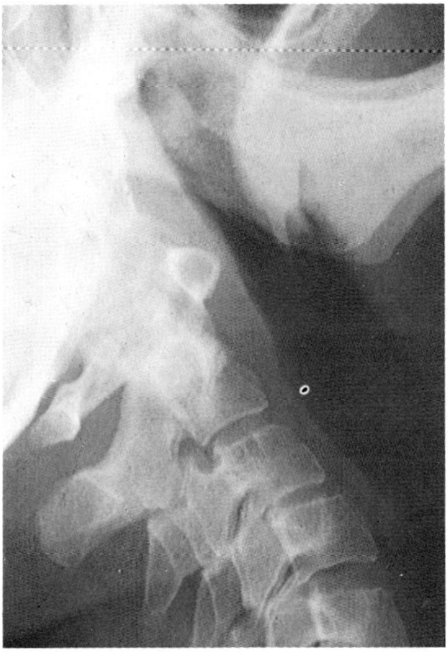

26

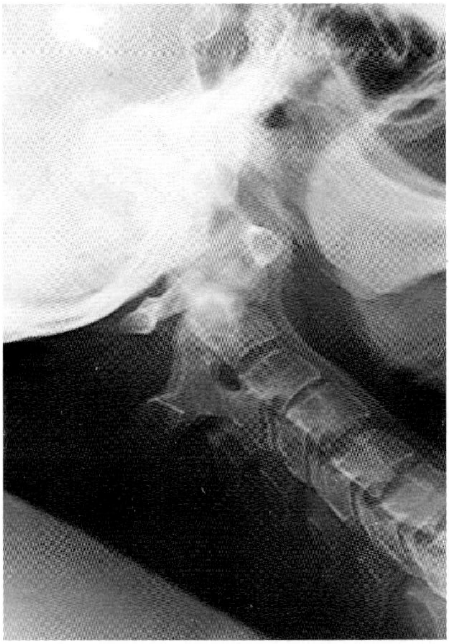

25 Cervical spine is the only segment of the vertebral column which may be seriously involved in rheumatoid arthritis. X-rays taken in extension and in flexion are essential to demonstrate instability. This X-ray taken in extension shows thinning of the C3–4 disc, with some backward subluxation of C3 on C4. Note that the atlantoaxial joint appears normal in this view; the distance between the anterior edge of the odontoid and the posterior edge of the arch of the atlas does not exceed the normal 3mm.

26 Flexion position the same patient (**25**). Gross instability of the atlanto-axial joint is now seen, as the distance between the anterior border of the odontoid and the posterior arch of the atlas has increased to 8mm. Instability of any segment of the cervical spine may lead to cord compression with consequent myelopathy, usually a spastic tetraparesis. Multiradicular lower motor neurone signs may also be present in the arms.

27

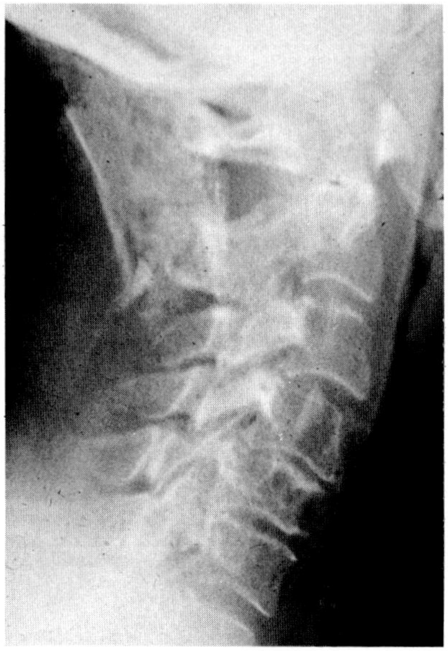

27 Rheumatoid arthritis of the lower cervical spine with partial destruction of the discs between C4–5 and C5–6. Note the absence of osteophytes and erosion of the upper border of C5, features which distinguish this condition from cervical spondylosis. Note also that this patient has had an occipitocervical fusion for atlantoaxial instability.

28 Advanced involvement of cervical spine with gross subluxation of C4 on C5, and destruction of the disc between C5 and C6.

29 Myelogram of the same patient (**28**) showing blockage at the same level.

30 Autopsy specimen of a patient who died from the consequences of cervical cord compression due to rheumatoid arthritis. Note major compression of the cervical cord at C4–5 level. Quite severe atlantoaxial subluxation may occur in the absence of a myelopathy, whereas minor degrees of subluxation at lower levels may compress the cord. This is because the cervical canal widens appreciably above the body of C2, as can be well seen in this illustration.

28

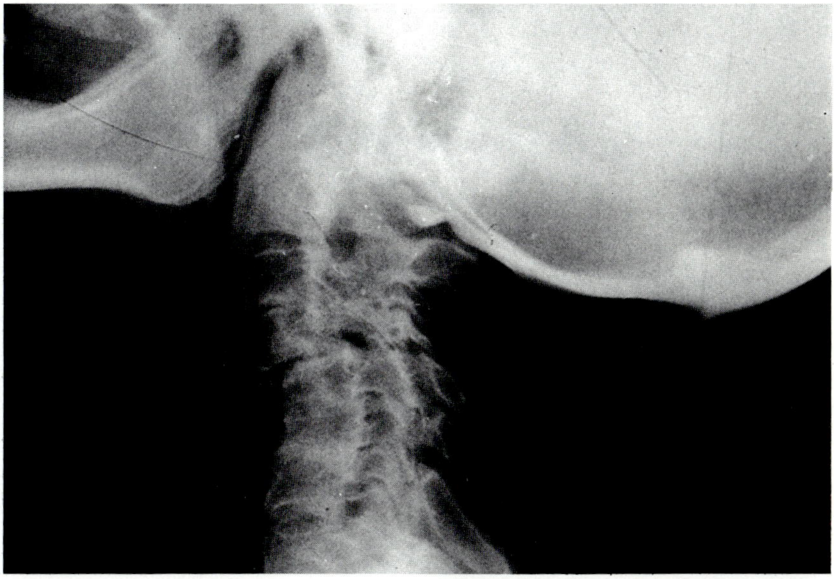

29

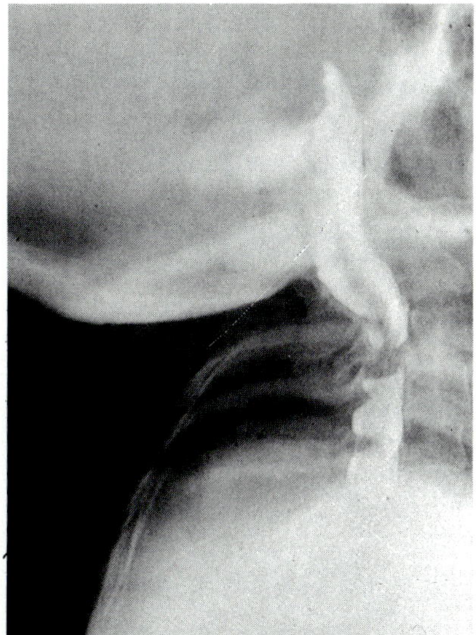

30

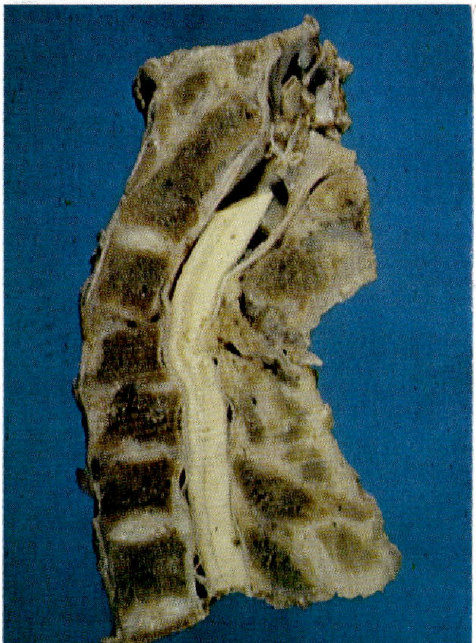

31

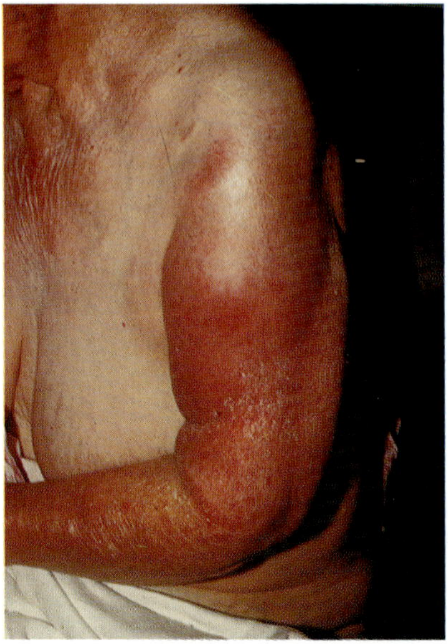

32

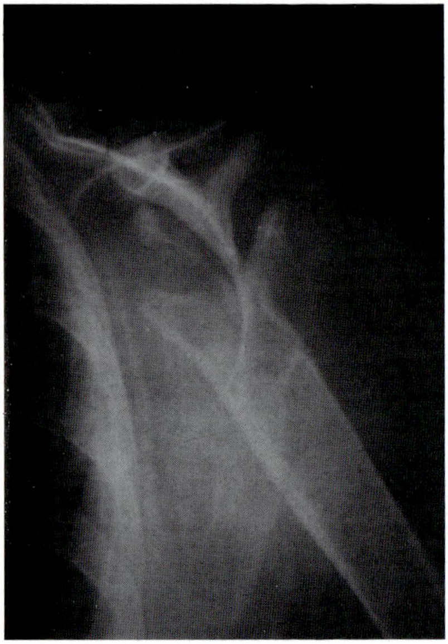

31 Pyarthrosis of the shoulder. Joints affected by rheumatoid arthritis are unduly susceptible to infection – frequently by the staphylococcus. An unwary clinician may accept a sudden exacerbation of pain and swelling to be due to an increase in rheumatoid activity within the joint if this is not borne in mind. Early diagnosis of a pyarthrosis is essential, since destructive changes occur with alarming rapidity, and in addition the condition may be life threatening. Any rheumatoid joint presenting with unusually severe inflammatory signs should be suspected of being infected, and aspirated fluid sent for bacteriological examination. Accompanying systemic signs, such as fever and leucocytosis should be looked for. This illustration shows such a condition, and pus has already tracked down the upper arm.

32 Severe destructive changes resulting from a pyarthrosis. Three weeks after onset almost total destruction of the humeral head and glenoid have occured.

33

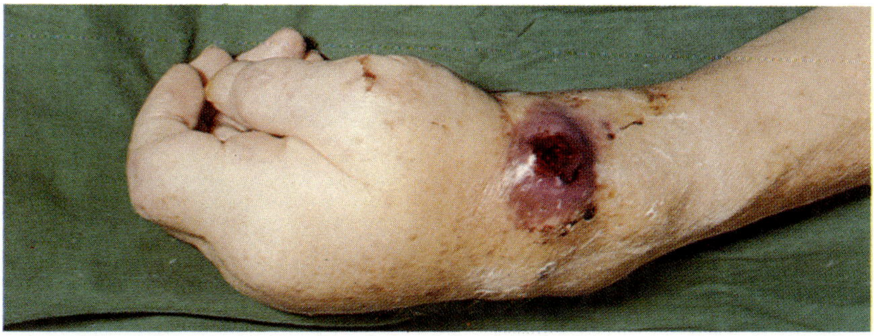

33 Pyarthrosis complicating rheumatoid arthritis of the wrist joint. A few weeks before, the patient had presented with an infected penetrating ulcer on the foot.

34

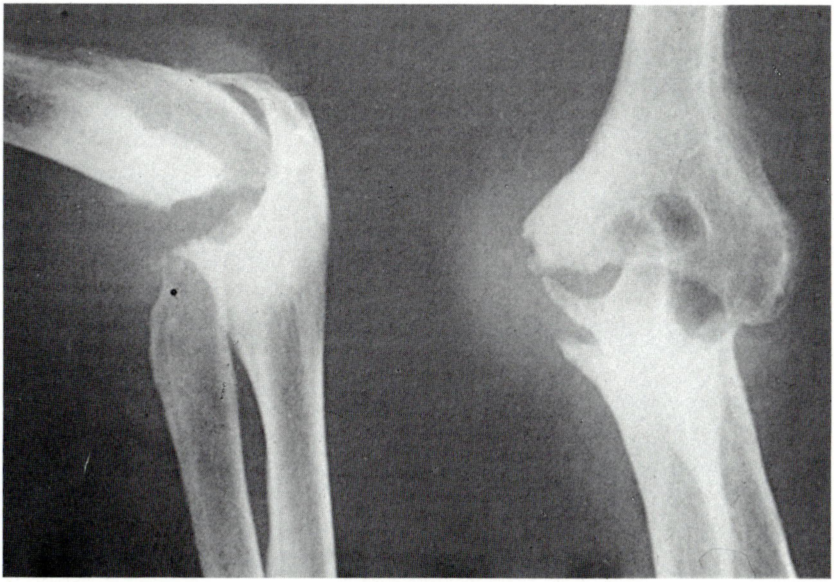

34 Pyarthrosis of the elbow joint complicating rheumatoid arthritis. Again gross destructive changes are shown.

35

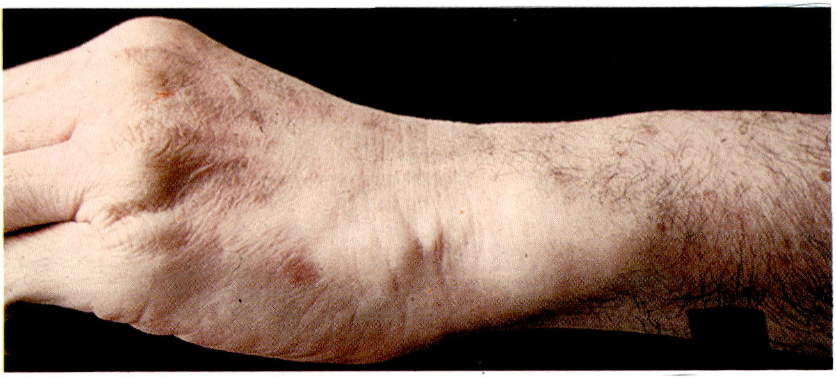

35 Tendons and their sheaths may be involved by effusion or nodule formation. Tendon sheath swelling due to tenosynovitis is common. An effusion is seen in the sheath overlying the end of the ulna.

36

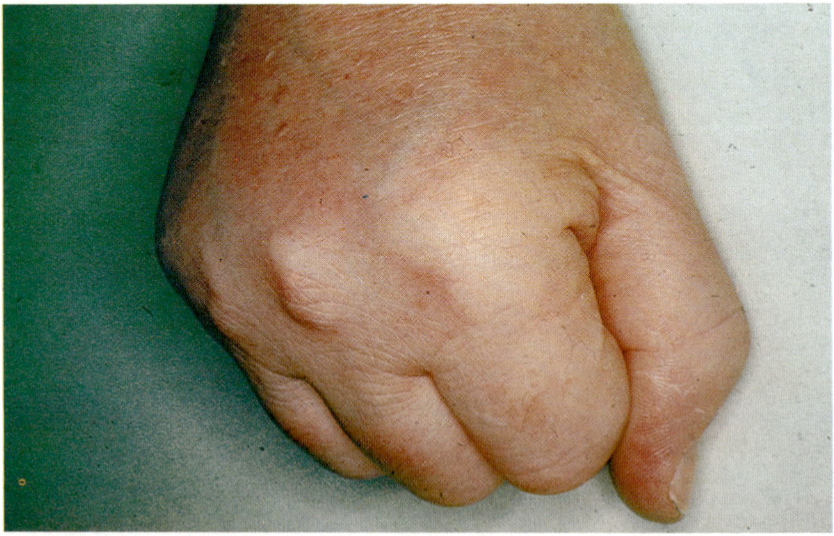

36 Nodule formation in the tendon of extensor digitorum longus. Nodules in finger flexor tendons are more usual and may cause triggering of the fingers, especially in the early morning.

37

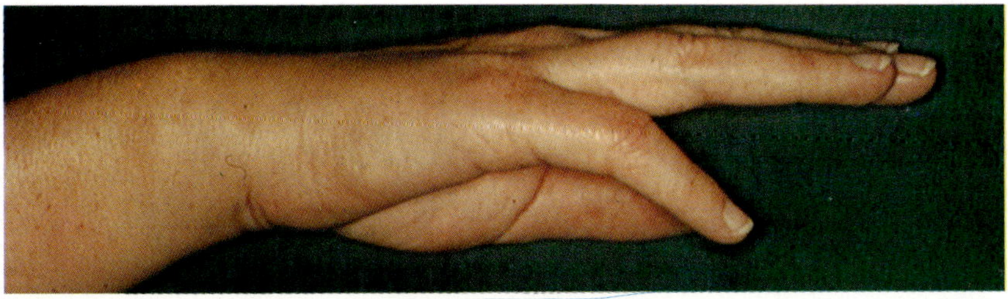

37 Attrition rupture of tendons (usually extensor tendons) may occur suddenly, and be due to quite minor strain. Two causes are apparent: (1) softening of the tendon due to inflammatory tendinitis; (2) attrition of the tendon due to subluxation at the wrist joint, the tendon riding over roughened bone surfaces.

38

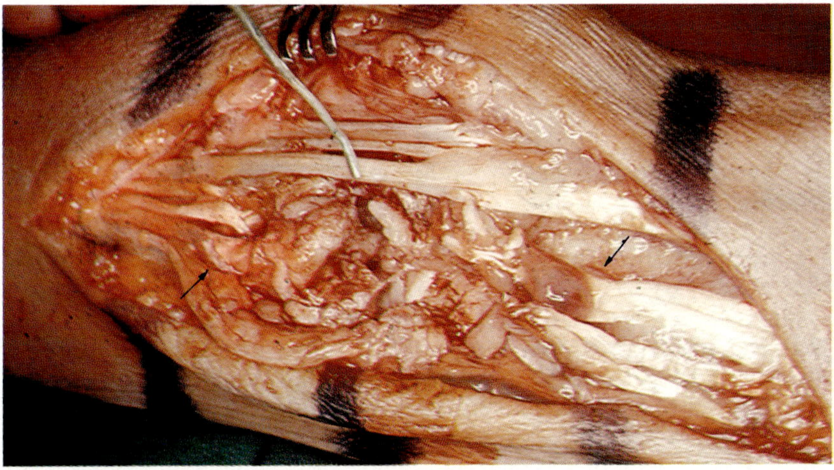

38 Rupture of two extensor tendons. The widely separated ends of the two ruptured tendons (*arrowed*) are seen in the lower half of the illustration, indicating the difficulty which may be experienced in obtaining apposition at operation. The upper tendons are intact and the probe points to a roughened spicule of bone held to be partially responsible for the attrition of the ruptured tendons. Surgical aid should be sought early, since wide separation of the tendons may make repair impossible.

39

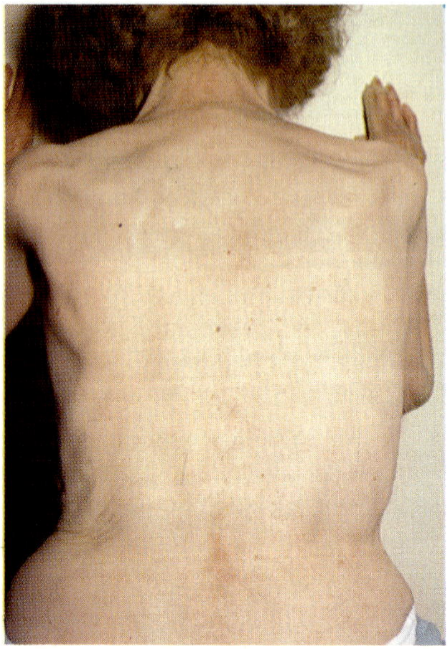

40

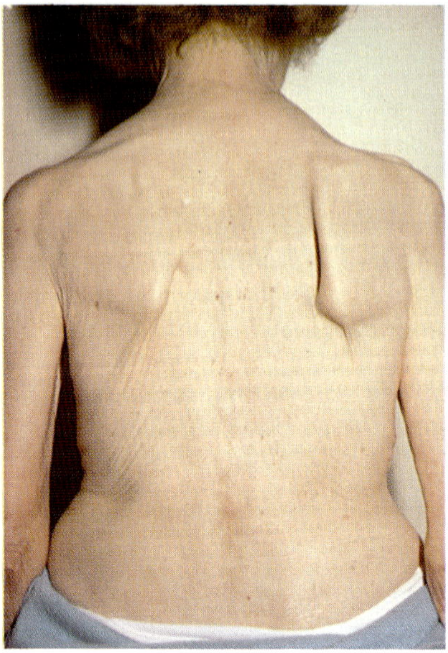

39 Proximal rheumatoid myopathy of the shoulder girdle with profound wasting of the supra- and infra- spinati. Such a proximal myopathy may occur as an integral part of rheumatoid arthritis, most commonly affecting the shoulder girdle. Diagnosis may be difficult since the muscles may already be severely wasted secondary to involvement of the shoulder joints themselves. In addition weakness, giving rise to inability to raise the arms may be wrongly interpreted as restriction due to pain. Treatment with steroids may also cause a proximal myopathy, and distinguishing between the two causes may present a diagnostic problem.

40 Posterior view of another patient showing in addition marked winging of the right scapula.

41

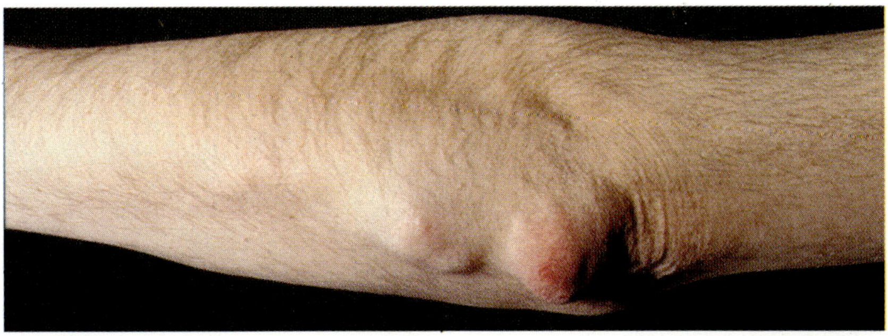

41 Skin nodules occur in about 25% of patients with rheumatoid arthritis. They are usually associated with severe disease and a high titre of rheumatoid factor and generally indicate a poor prognosis. The elbow is their most common site, where they may be single or multiple. In addition inflammation may affect the olecranon bursa. This picture shows both a skin nodule and an enlarged and inflamed olecranon bursa.

42

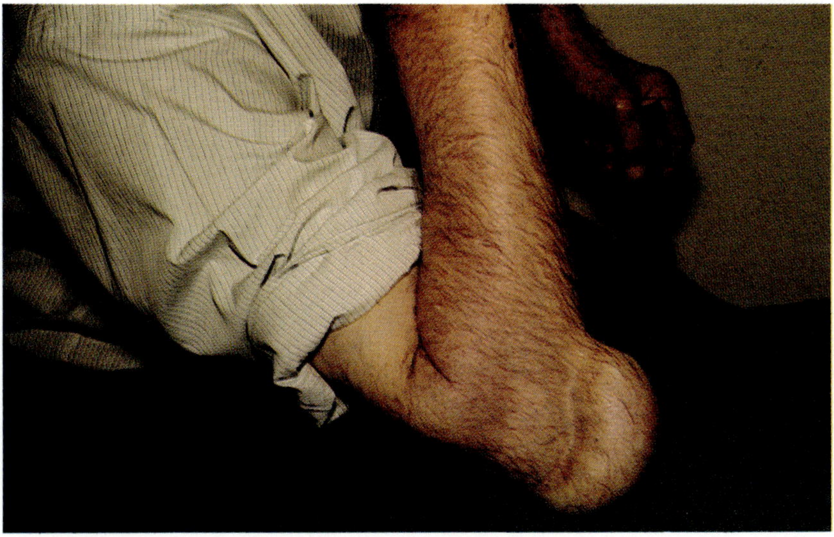

42 Solitary massive enlargement of the olecranon bursa. A similar condition may be seen in chronic gout (see **162**).

43

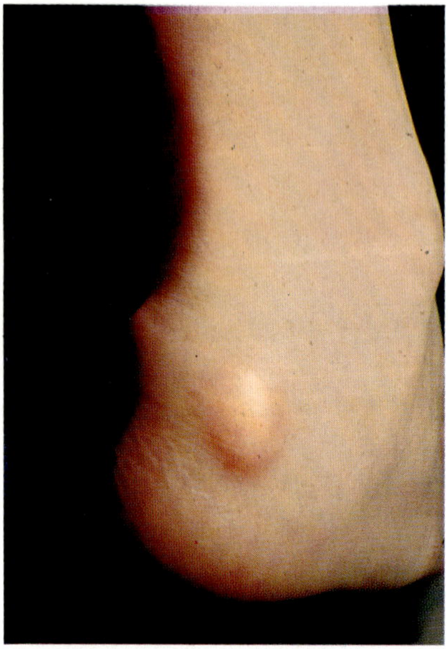

44

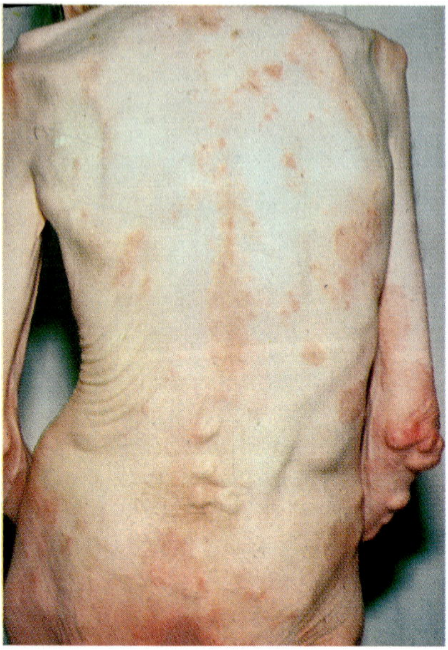

43 The Achilles tendon is another common site of nodule formation.

44 Skin nodules over the back of the sacrum and on both elbows. In patients confined to bed, these frequently break down causing pressure sores.

45 Deeply perforating ulcers on the feet may occur due to relative ischaemia and pressure on nodules or over subluxed joints.

46 Ulcers on the lower leg are common and probably have a multiple aetiology. The skin in rheumatoid arthritis is thin and atrophic and easily damaged, while the peripheral circulation is poor due to stasis. Some of these ulcers may also have an arteritic basis (see section on cardiovascular complications).

47 Severe gold dermatitis. Rashes are not a feature of adult rheumatoid arthritis, though they may occur in some types of juvenile chronic arthritis (see page 60). Drug eruptions are, however, not uncommon as a complication of treatment, notably with gold compounds (of which this is an example), D-penicillamine and others.

45

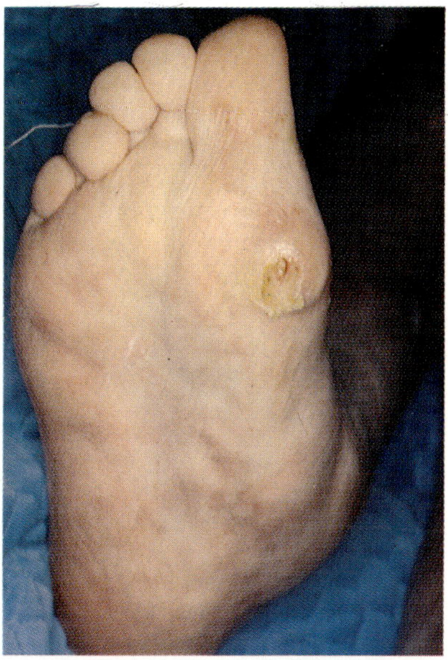

46

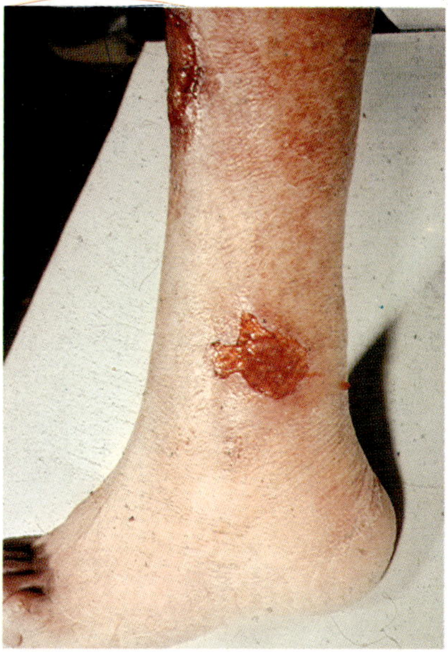

47

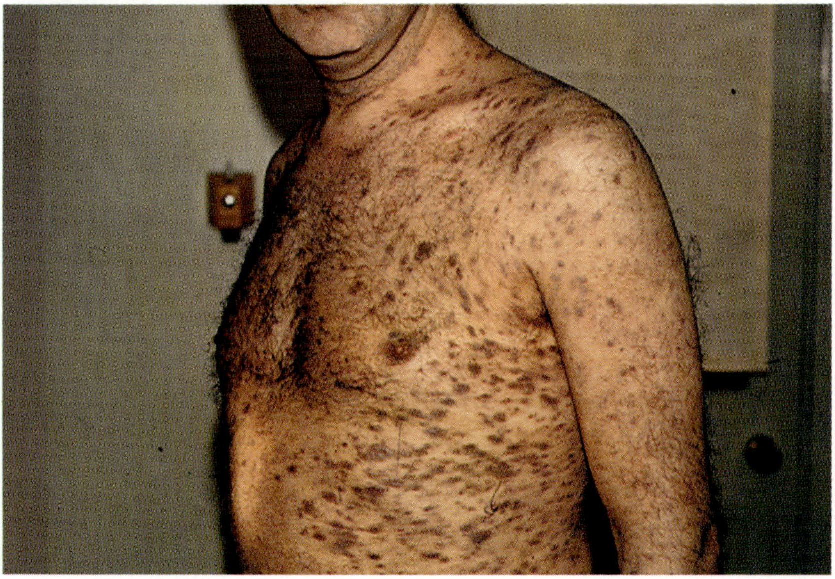

48 Rheumatoid episcleritis. This is a common ocular complication of rheumatoid arthritis and generally indicates a poor prognosis. It is often associated with skin nodules, a high titre of rheumatoid factor, and sometimes vasculitis. The incidence of iritis in rheumatoid arthritis is no greater than that found in the general population.

49 Rheumatoid scleritis is more serious and may eventually lead to involvement of the whole uveal tract with risk of eventual glaucoma. Blue discolouration of the sclera may eventually occur.

50 Nodular scleritis is a more advanced stage of the previous case.

48

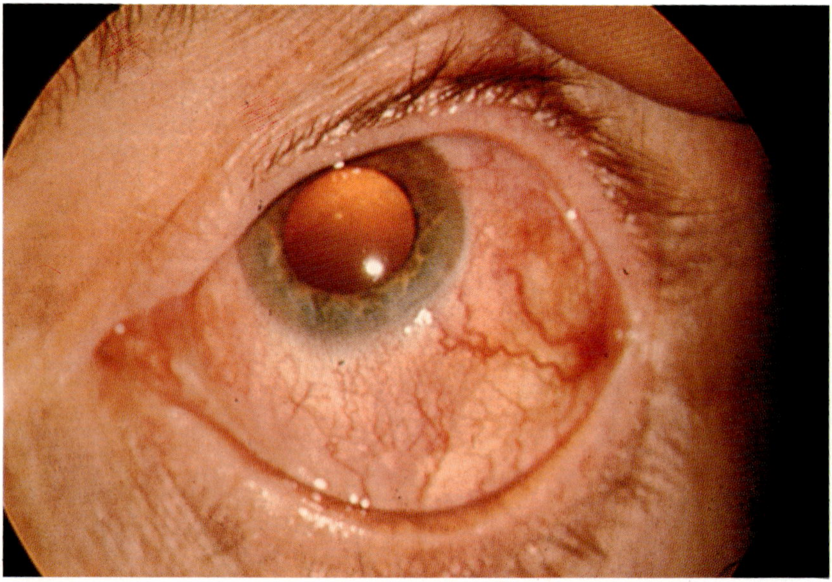

49

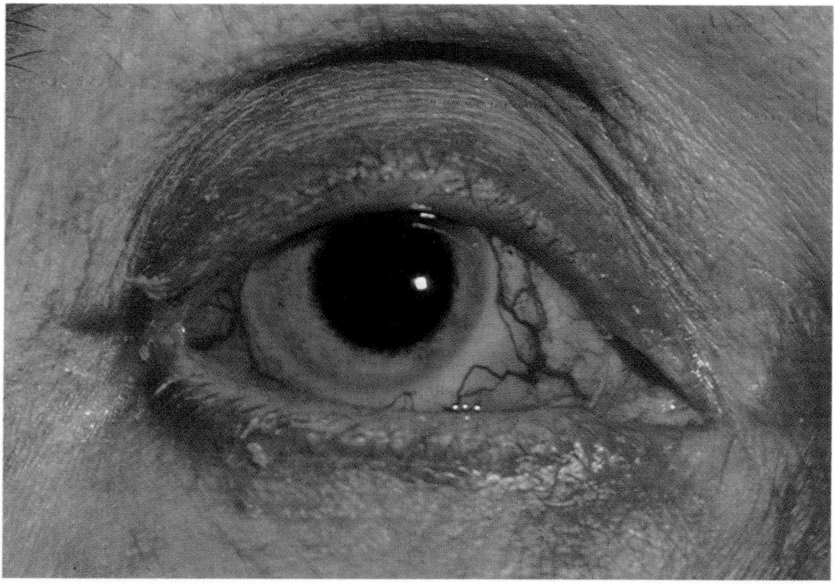

50

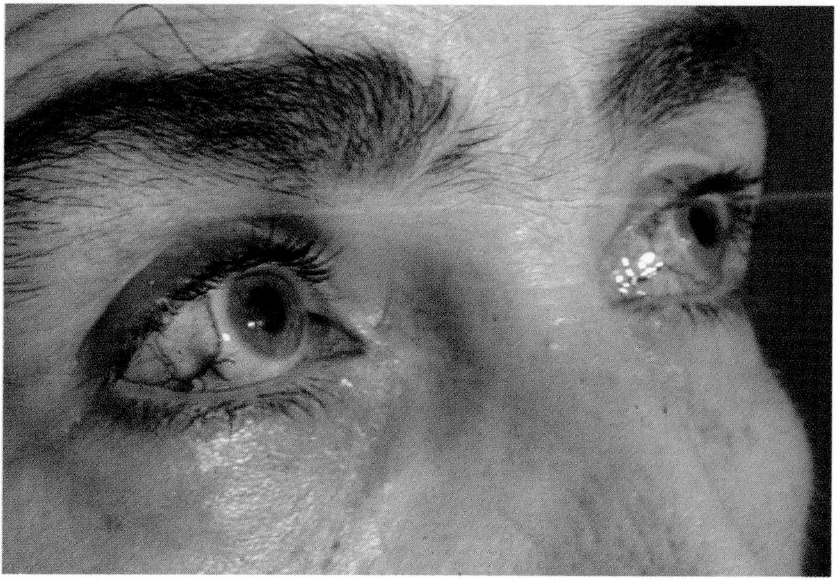

51 Scleromalacia perforans. At a later stage nodules which have formed in the sclera may break down giving rise to ulceration. As with scleritis, this is usually associated with severe disease, skin nodules and vasculitis and carries a poor prognosis.

52 Sjögren's syndrome is manifested by keratoconjunctivitis sicca and a severe rheumatoid arthritis. Dryness of the eyes and mouth is characteristic, and lack of bronchial secretion and atrophic gastritis may occur. Deficient lachrymal secretion may be tested for by Schirmer's test, but staining with Rose Bengal is more reliable. Tiny superficial ulcers take up the stain as shown here. Keratoconjunctivitis sicca may also occur in other connective tissue disorders, notably progressive systemic sclerosis.

53 Posterior subcapsular cataracts may occur particularly after prolonged steroid therapy. Steroids may also precipitate the onset of glaucoma.

51

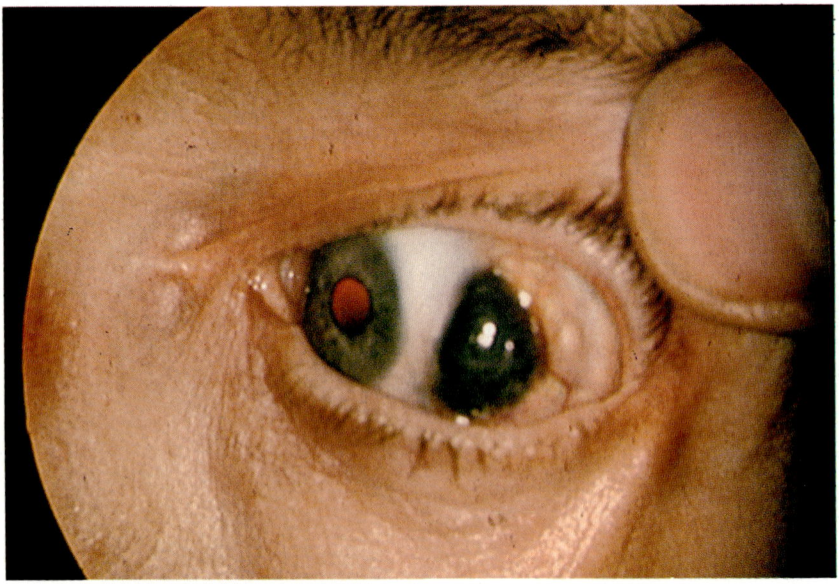

52

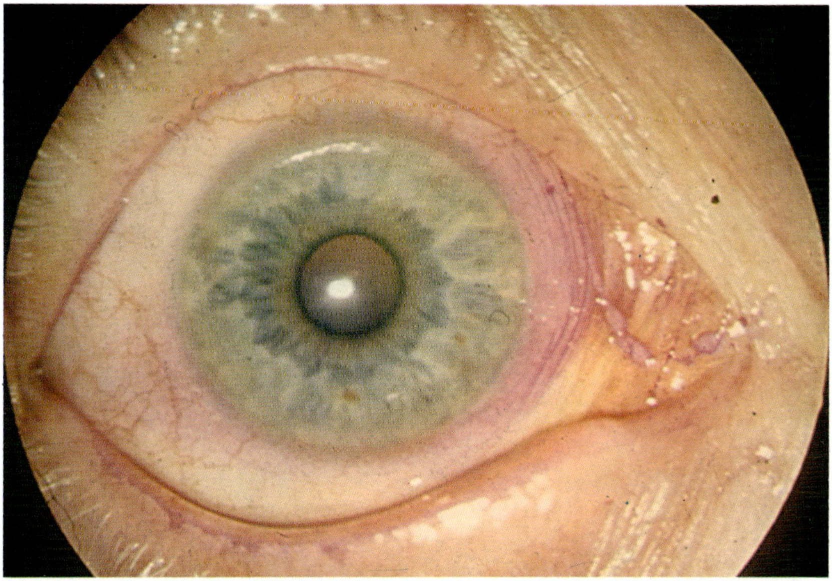

53

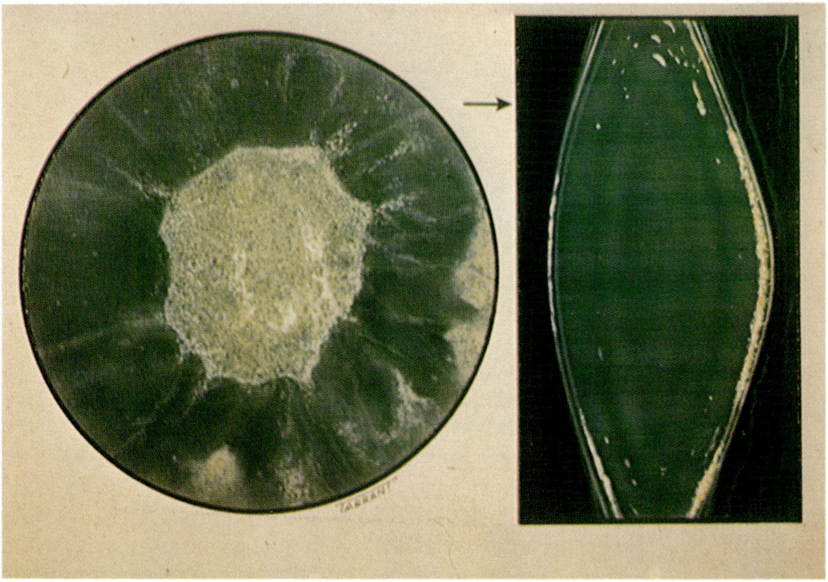

54

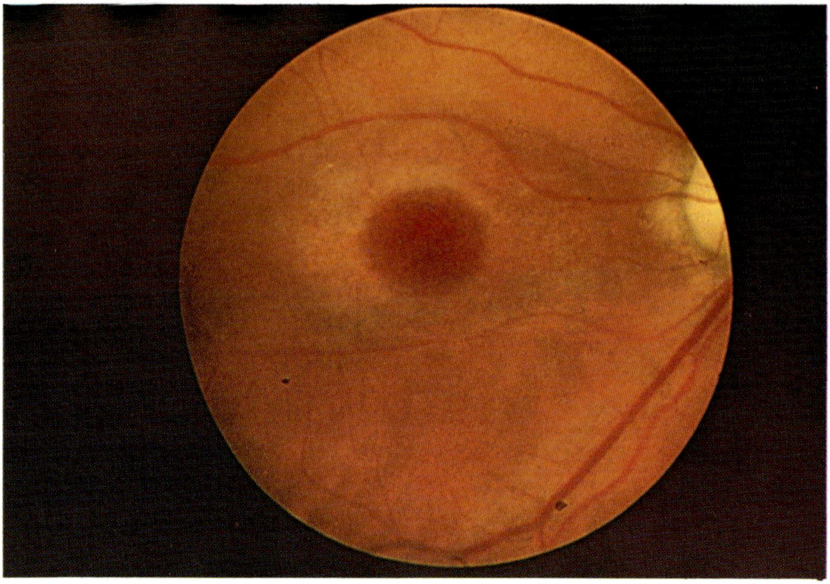

54 Chloroquine retinopathy. Another serious eye complaint may be induced by prolonged treatment with anti-malarial drugs. This is a Chloroquine retinopathy showing the typical 'bull's eye' formation, with atrophy of retinal cells.

The lungs

55 Solitary lung nodule in the 4th right interspace. Rheumatoid nodules may be present in the lung parenchyema or in the pleura. They may be single or multiple. Differential diagnosis from other round shadows in the lung (e.g. carcinoma) may be difficult.

56 Tomogram of previous X-ray. Note that cavitation has occurred in the central part of the nodule.

57 Rheumatoid pleural effusions may be unilateral or bilateral, and typically occur in the middle aged male. These effusions (unless large or bilateral or both) are often symptomless, and many of them resolve spontaneously. Diagnosis may be aided by the fact that a positive test for rheumatoid factor may be found in the fluid aspirated for examination.

55

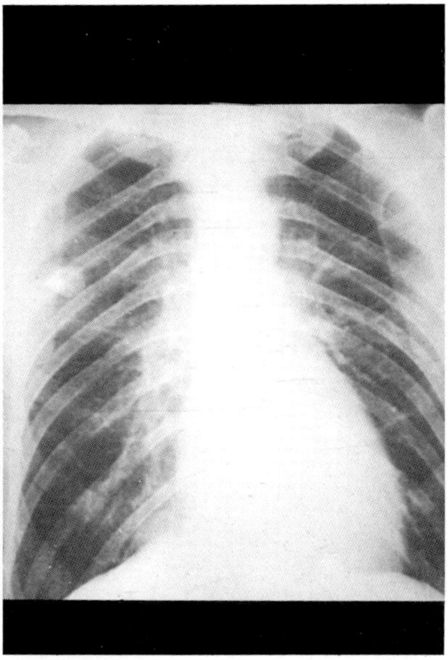

56

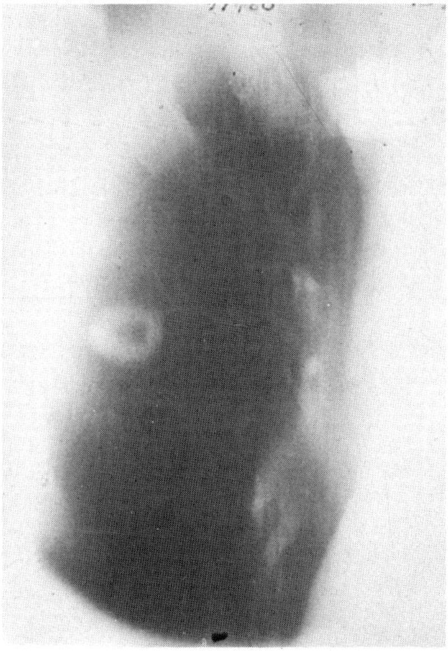

57

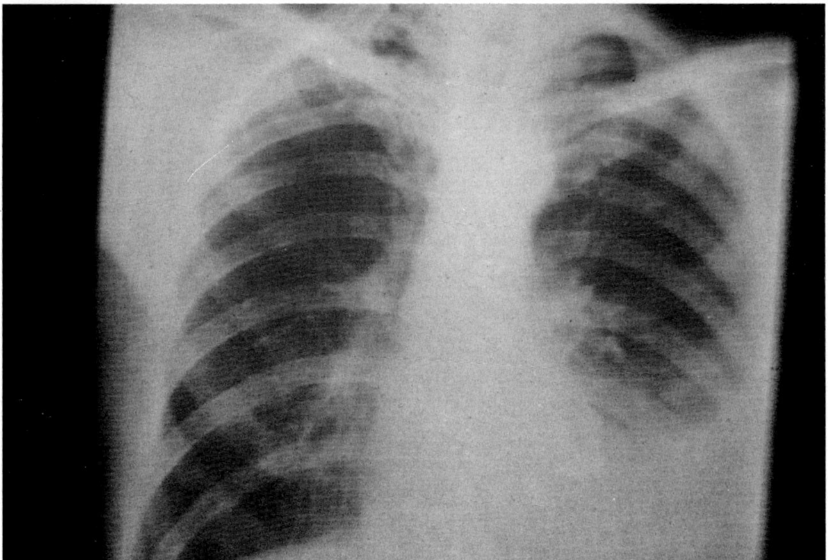

58 The rheumatoid lung. This is a fibrosing alveolitis, at first confined to the basal areas, but may eventually involve the whole lung field. Fibrosing alveolitis may occur without other manifestations of rheumatoid arthritis, but many such patients show a positive test for rheumatoid factor. In a proportion of these patients true rheumatoid arthritis may eventually develop after the lapse of months or even years.

59 Fibrosing alveolitis well seen at the right base, with early changes in the upper lung fields.

60 Rheumatoid lung may be associated with clubbing of the fingers in addition to the stigmata of rheumatoid arthritis as illustrated.

58

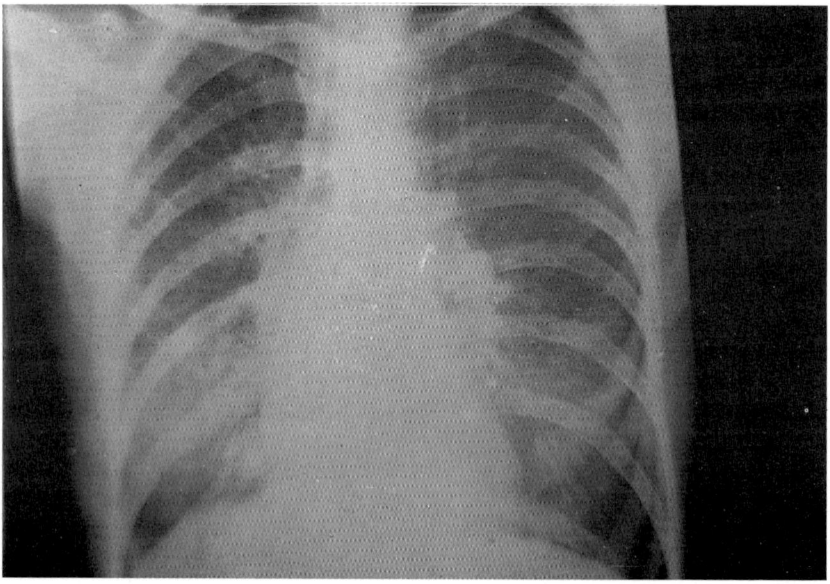

59

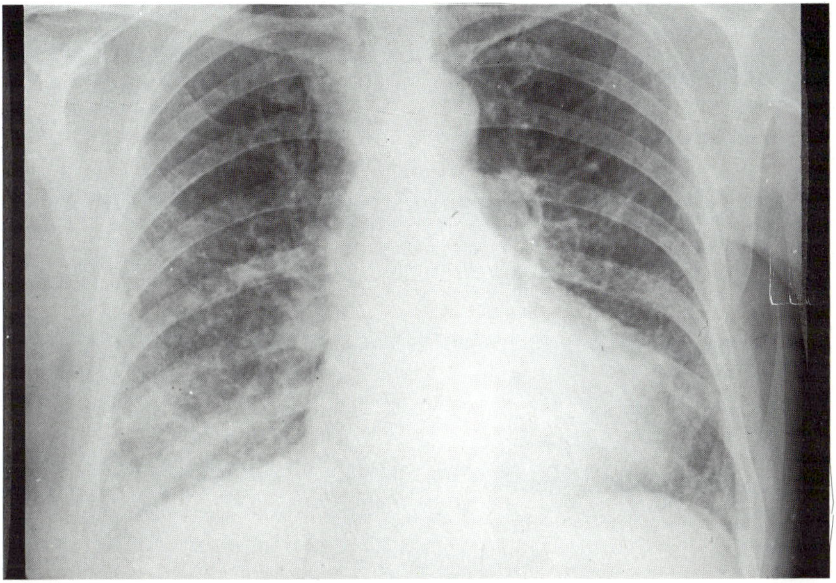

60

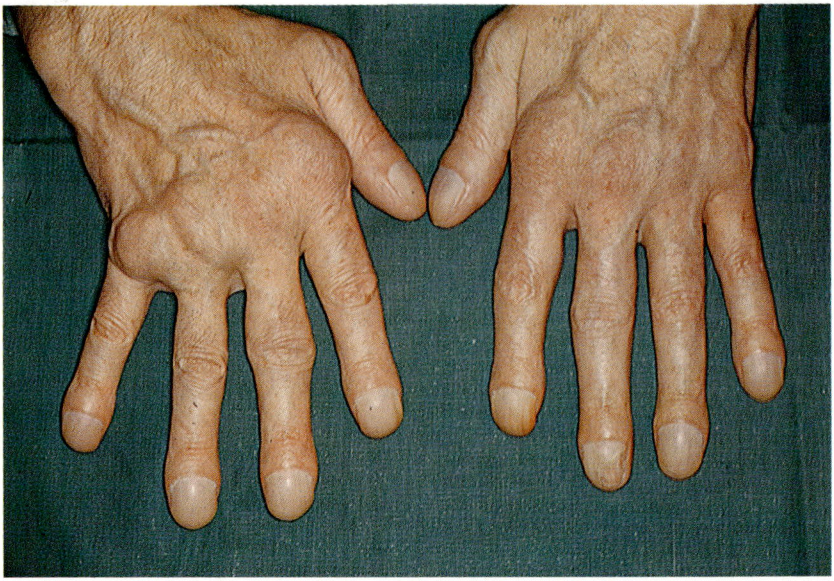

61

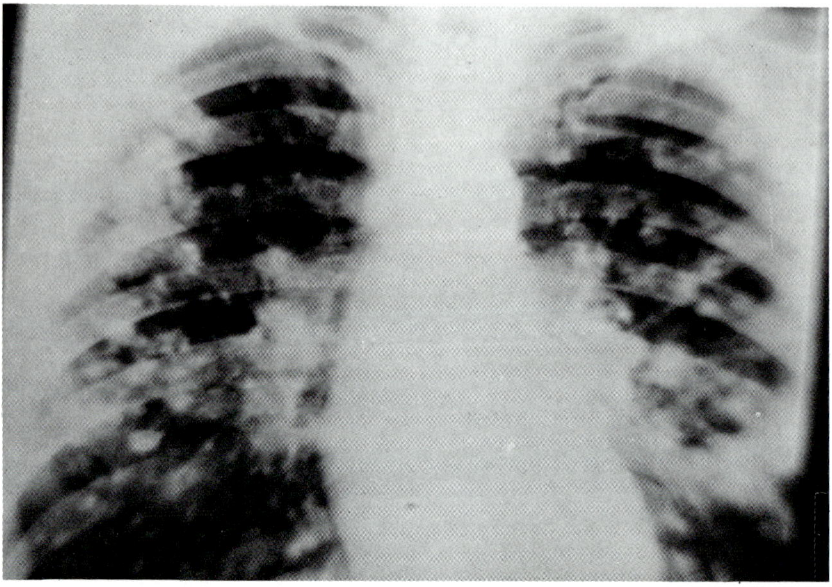

62

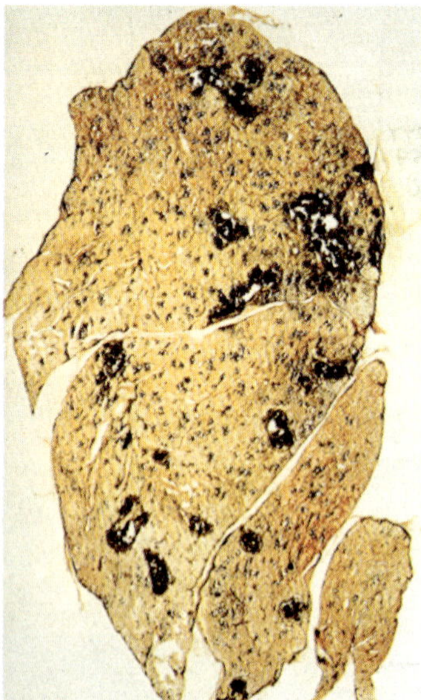

61 Caplan's syndrome occurs in about 35% of coal miners who have rheumatoid arthritis, and is manifested by discrete nodules measuring more than 1cm in diameter throughout the lung fields, and superimposed on a background of pneumoconiosis. As with fibrosing alveolitis, these changes may precede the development of the arthropathy. A similar condition may occur in those who work with asbestos, silica, and other abrasive dusts.

62 Caplan's syndrome. Autopsy appearance of the lung.

63

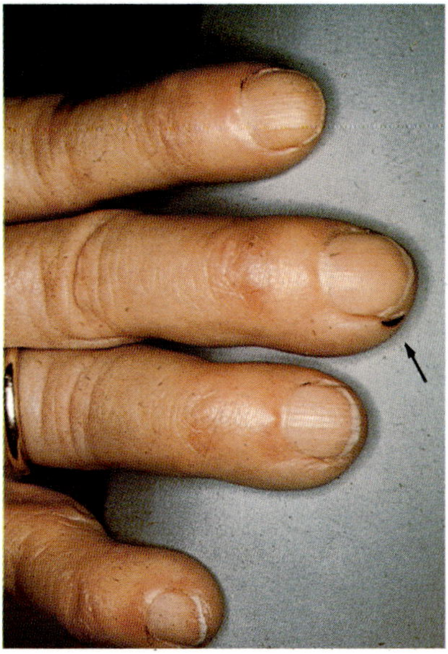

64

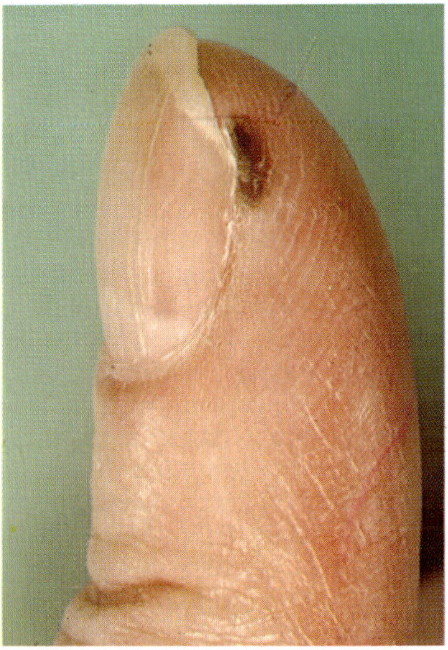

63 Nail fold lesions are an expression of digital arteritis due to inflammation, and eventual thrombosis of the tiny end-arteries. The lesion on the ulnar side of the middle finger is typical (*arrowed*). Minor lesions are also seen on the nail bed of the index and little fingers. Digital arteritis may be benign and self-limiting, or may be premonitory of an ensuing generalised rheumatoid vasculitis. Measurement of complement levels may be helpful in distinguishing between the two conditions, since in benign digital arteritis they are usually normal, whereas the level of C3 is reduced in the more generalised form.

64 Digital arteritis. Close up view of a typical nail fold lesion.

65 More advanced arteritic lesions involving not only the nail folds, but also seen over both 3rd metacarpophalangeal joints.

66 More advanced peripheral arterial lesions indicating involvement of larger vessels, and leading to gangrene of the digits. This usually heralds a fatal outcome for the patient since it is likely that the condition is widespread, involving the arterial system of all organs of the body. In such patients there is a significant mortality from ischaemic heart disease, cerebrovascular accidents, or multiple gut perforations. Peripheral neuropathy is also a common neurological complication (see page 54).

65

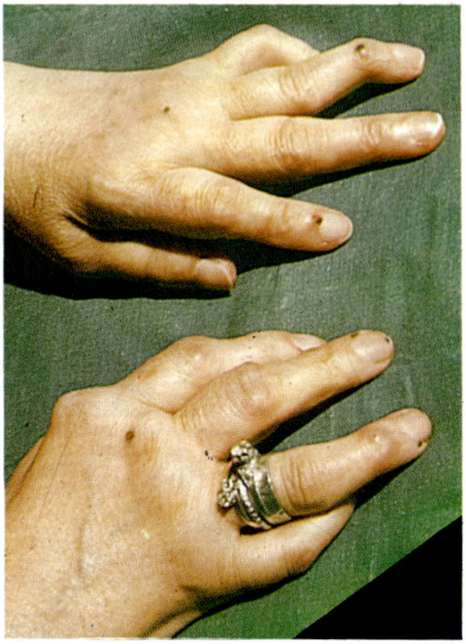

66

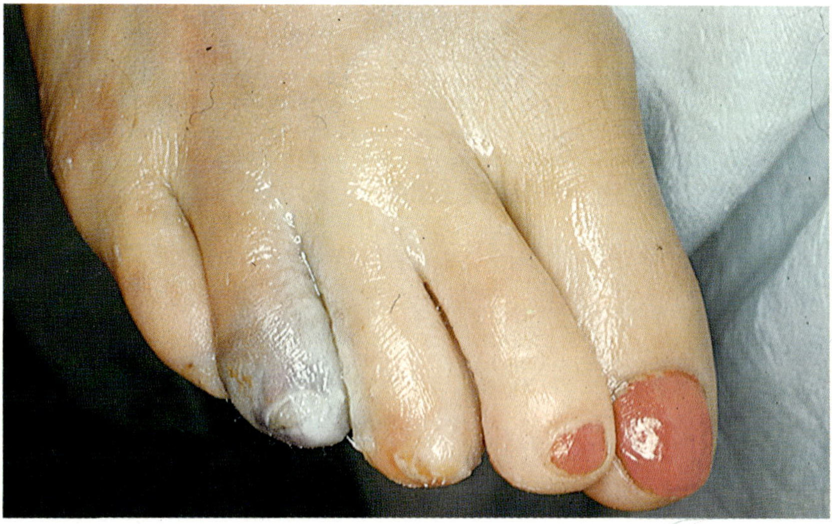

67

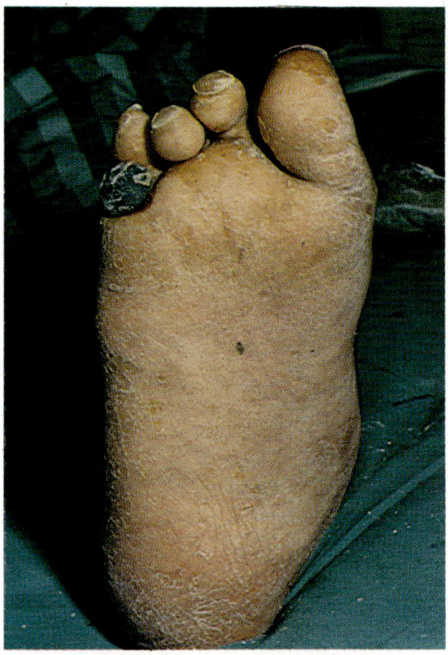

67 Dry gangrene of the 5th toe due to rheumatoid vasculitis.

68 Multiple small cardiac infarcts due to rheumatoid vasculitis.

68

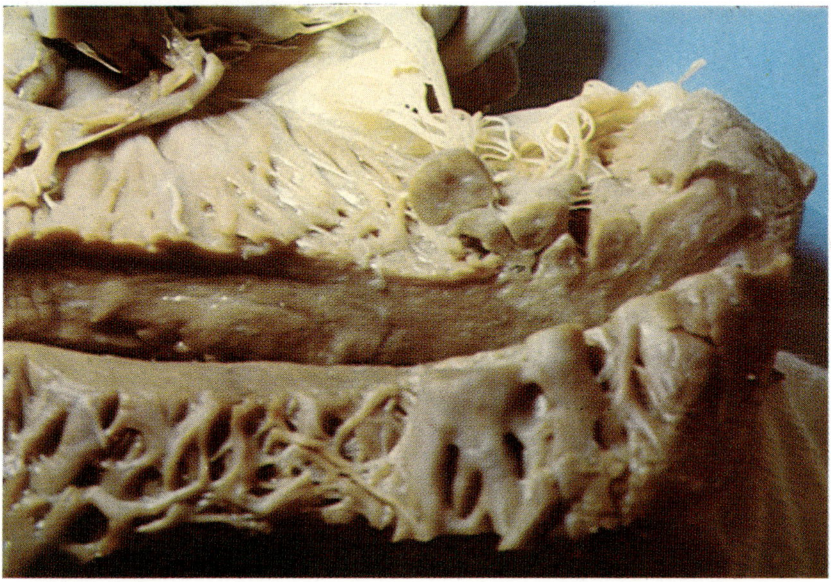

69 Perforation of the stomach (*arrowed*) due to arteritis involving the blood supply to the gut.

70 Splenic infarction due to arteritis involving the blood supply to the gut.

71 Vasculitis. An inflammation of the intima of the small and medium sized vessels, with round cell infiltration, may proceed to thrombosis within the vessel. In benign cases the media and internal elastic lamina may remain intact. (× *50*)

72 Advanced arteritis. There is almost complete destruction of the intima of the vessel and thrombosis has occurred. (× *30*)

69

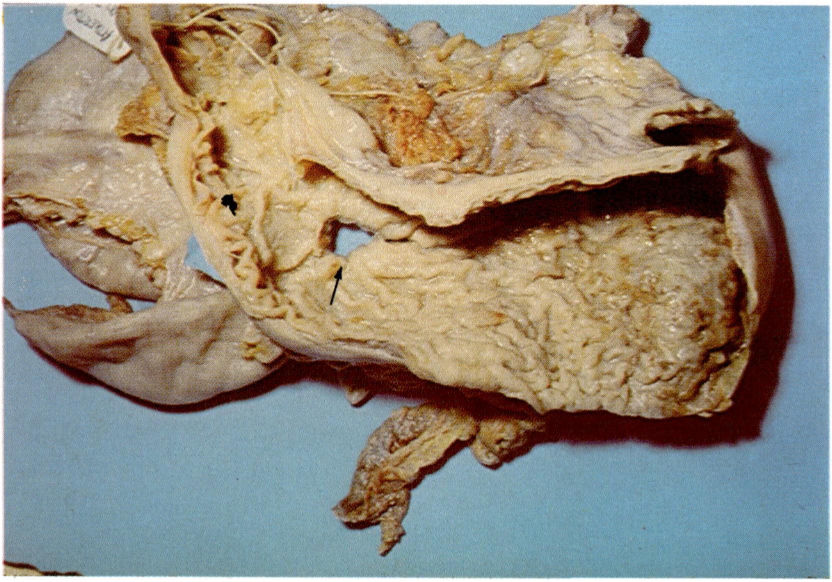

70

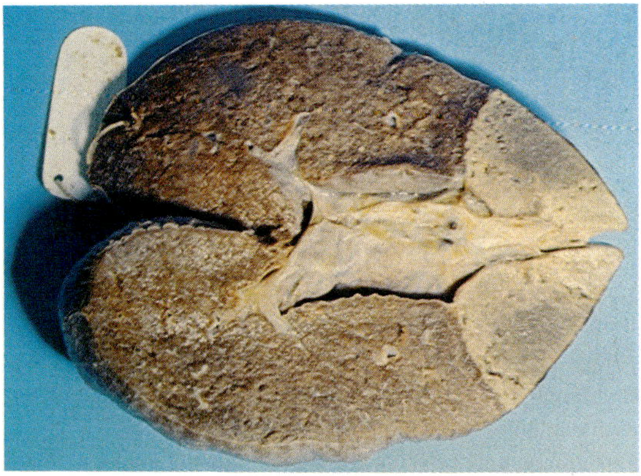

71

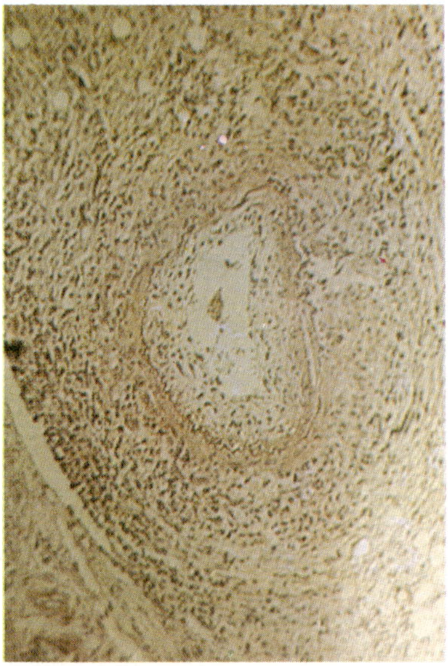

72

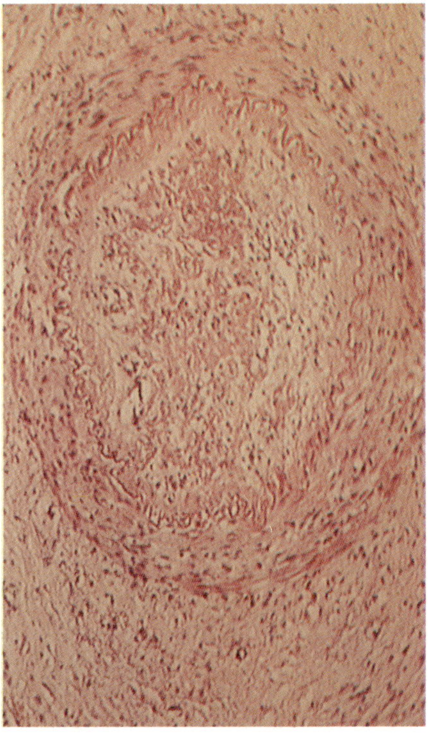

73 Rupture of the sinus of Valsalva, the result of intra-cardiac nodule formation. The patient died suddenly in acute cardiac failure. Clinically, cardiac lesions are rare in rheumatoid arthritis, although vulvular lesions, and especially symptomless pericarditis have been described.

74 ECG of cardiomyopathy. Flattening of all waves resembles changes seen in myxoedema and pericardial effusion. This is another rare condition in rheumatoid arthritis which may lead to arrhythmias or cardiac failure.

75 Renal amyloid. The glomerular capillaries are greatly thickened by amyloid deposition. Rheumatoid arthritis is the most important cause of secondary amyloid disease, with an incidence of about 16%. It may present with proteinuria or a nephrotic syndrome. The diagnosis is most readily made by a rectal biopsy. (× *150*)

73

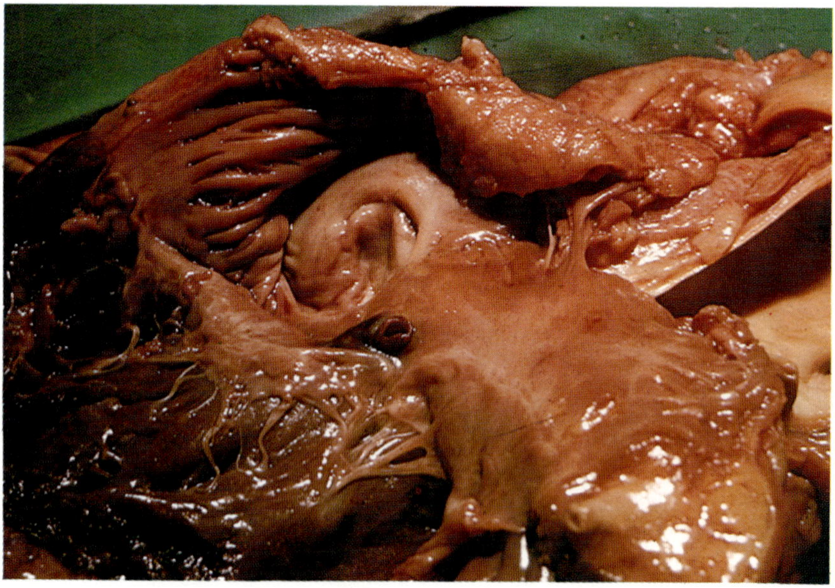

74

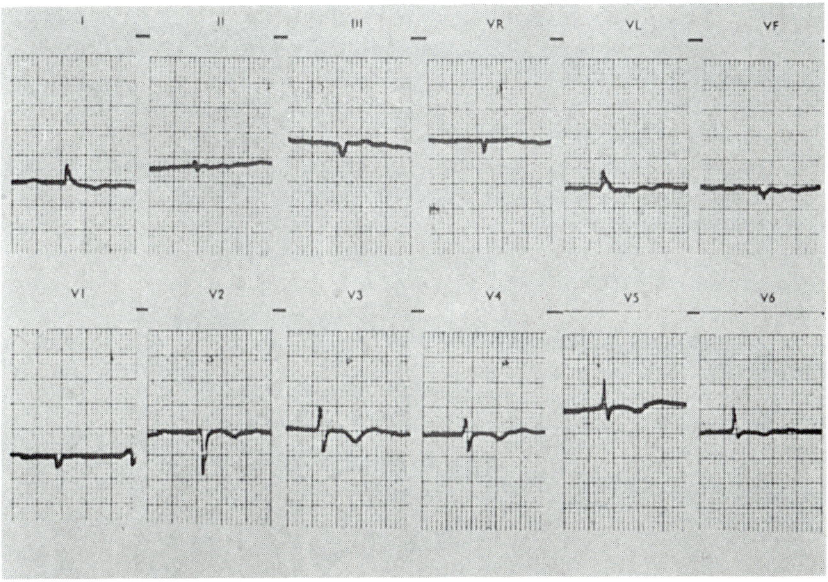

75

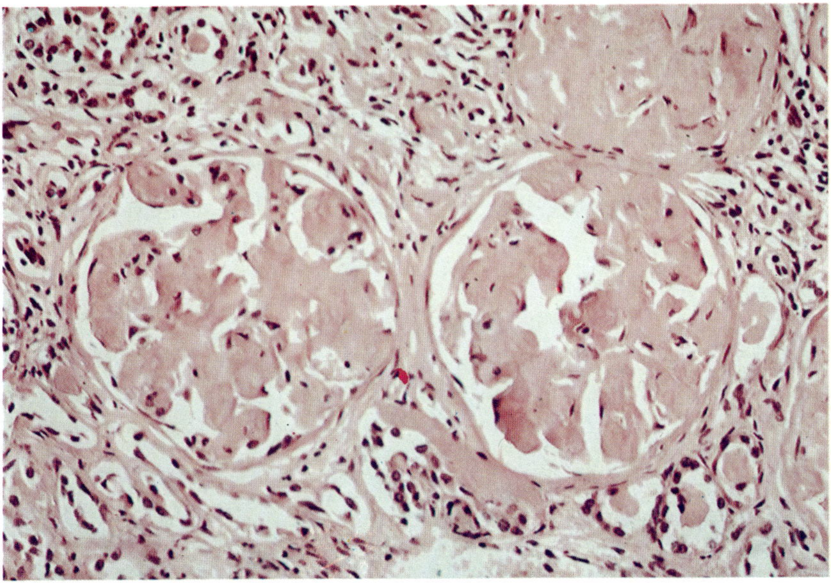

The nervous system

Involvement of the nervous system may be due to:
(a) entrapment neuropathies due to local pressure on peripheral nerves by swelling of neighbouring tissues involved in the inflammatory process, or from deformity of affected joints such as the elbow, which may cause compression of the ulnar nerve.
(b) interstitial neuropathy commonly presenting as a sensory neuropathy affecting the feet, but sometimes proceeding to a more severe sensorimotor neuropathy with a symmetrical distribution. Such cases usually occur in the presence of vasculitis in which the involvement of the vasa nervorum with consequent ischaemia of the nerve may be an aetiological factor.
(c) long tract compression of the spinal cord due to the involvement of the cervical spine (see **26–29**).

76 Wasting of the thenar eminences with sensory deficit over the median digits as a result of longstanding rheumatoid arthritis of the wrist joints, with consequent compression of the median nerves in the carpal tunnels. The carpal tunnel syndrome may be one of the earliest manifestations of rheumatoid arthritis, and if bilateral this diagnosis should always be borne in mind.

77 Bilateral peripheral neuropathy. The areas of sensory loss on the feet and lower legs is shown. Previous evidence of vasculitis is common in such patients, and the 'stocking' type anaesthesia may proceed to a mixed sensorimotor picture with foot drop.

78 Mixed sensorimotor neuropathy with unilateral foot drop. The prognosis in such patients is generally poor due to the associated vasculitis.

76

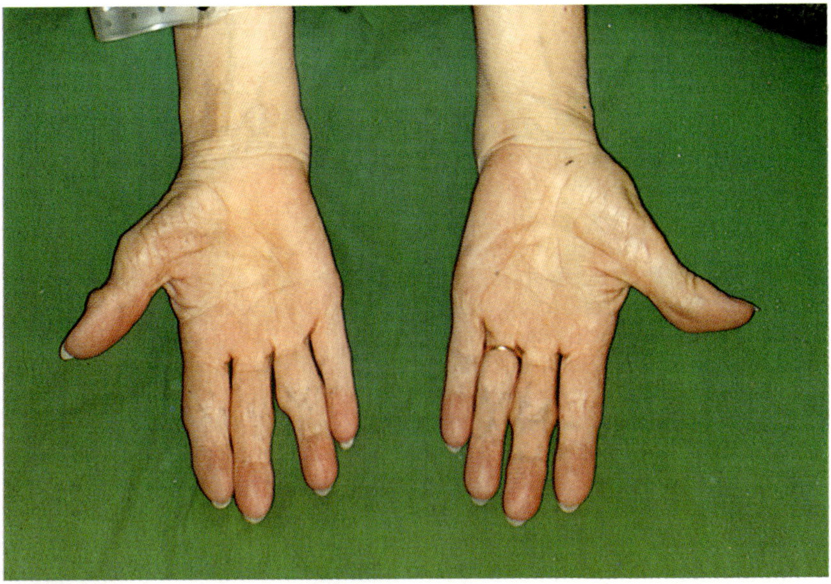

77

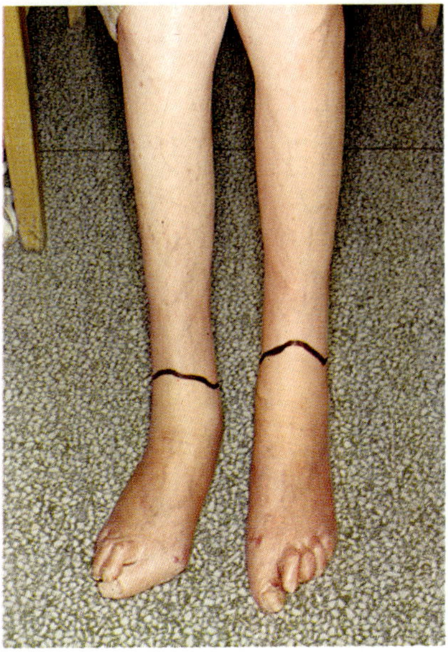

78

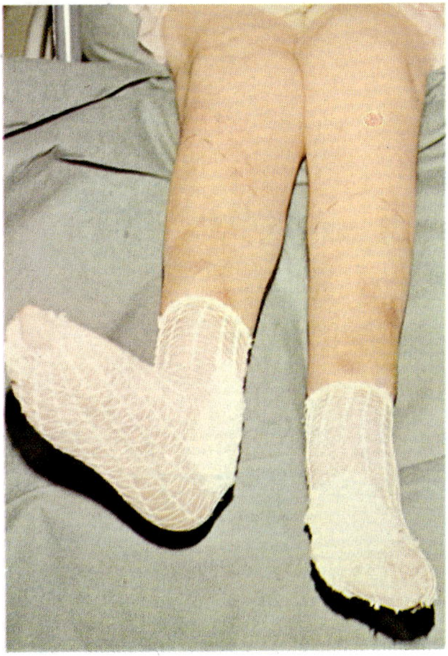

2 Juvenile chronic arthritis. (Still's disease)

Since the original description by Still in 1897, a number of subgroups of children suffering from arthritis have been identified as follows:

1 Still's disease with:
   (a) systemic manifestations
   (b) polyarticular disease
   (c) pauci-articular disease with or without chronic iridocyclitis
2 Adult type rheumatoid arthritis with IgM rheumatoid factor.
3 Juvenile ankylosing spondylitis.

Still's disease differs in certain respects from adult rheumatoid arthritis: (1) The arthritis is generally less destructive, but there is a marked tendency to involvement of the cervical spine: (2) fever at onset, rash, leucocytosis and lymphadenopathy with splenomegaly are common features: (3) nodules and rheumatoid factor are more often absent: (4) pericarditis may occur: and (5) iridocyclitis tends to occur in the pauci-articular form of the disease. Male children with arthritis of the knees and ankles may proceed in later years to involvement of the sacroiliac joints and spine, and show a higher than normal incidence of HLA–B27.

79

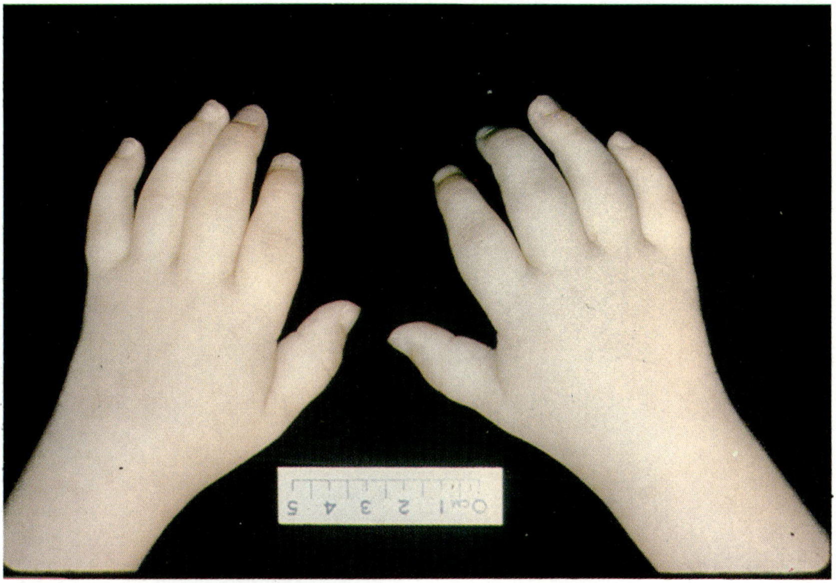

80

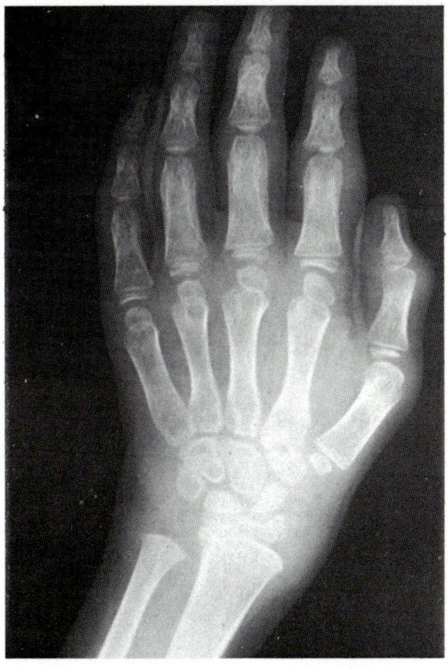

79 The hands in Still's disease showing marked swelling of the proximal interphalangeal joints.

80 Osteoporosis and marked soft tissue swelling shown in X-ray of the hand.

81 **82**

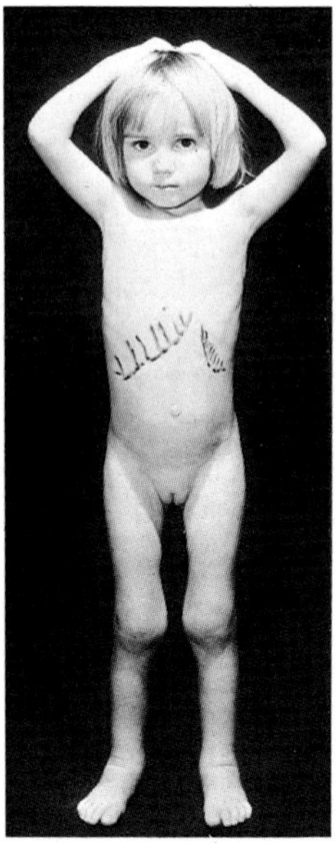

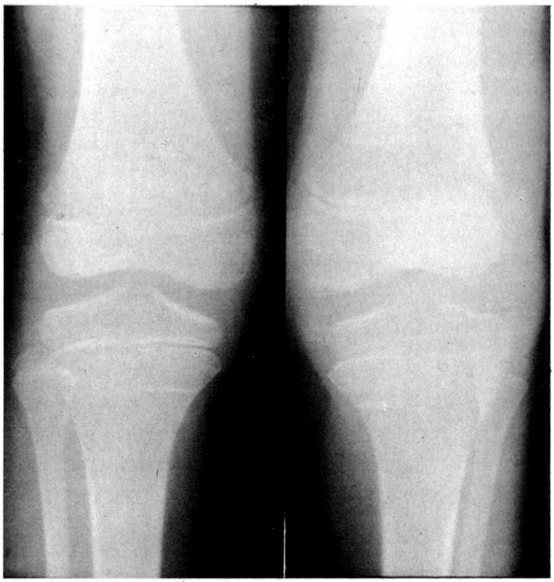

81 Still's disease showing marked swelling of both knees. The extent of splenic and liver enlargement have been marked on the skin.

82 Osteoporosis and soft tissue swelling of the right joint shown in X-ray of the knees.

83 Hip joints showing progressive changes over a 3-year period.

84 Ankylosis of the upper cervical spine shown in X-ray of the neck.

85 Temperature chart of early Still's disease. A high swinging fever is a common early manifestation.

83

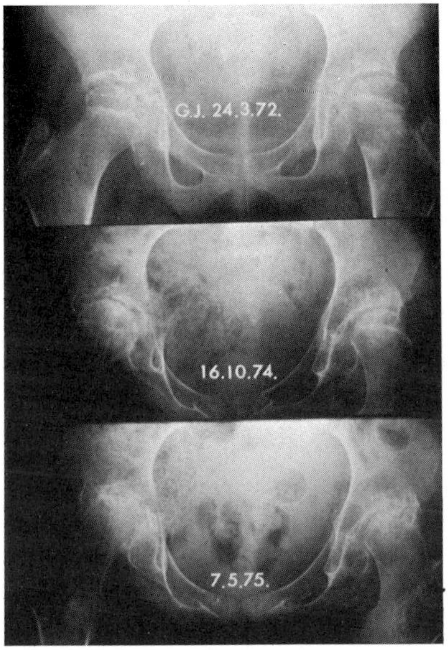
G.J. 24.3.72.
16.10.74.
7.5.75.

84

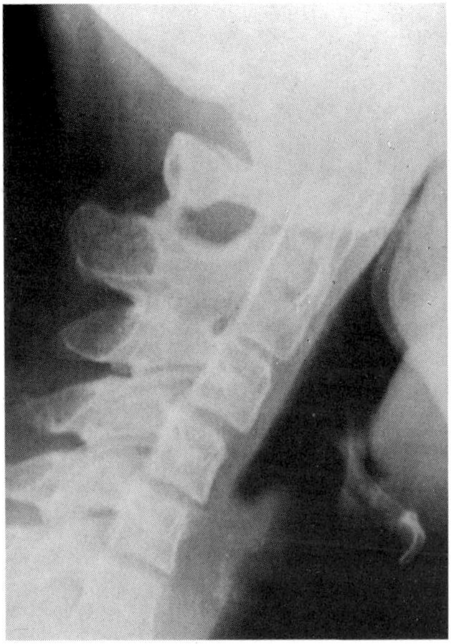

85

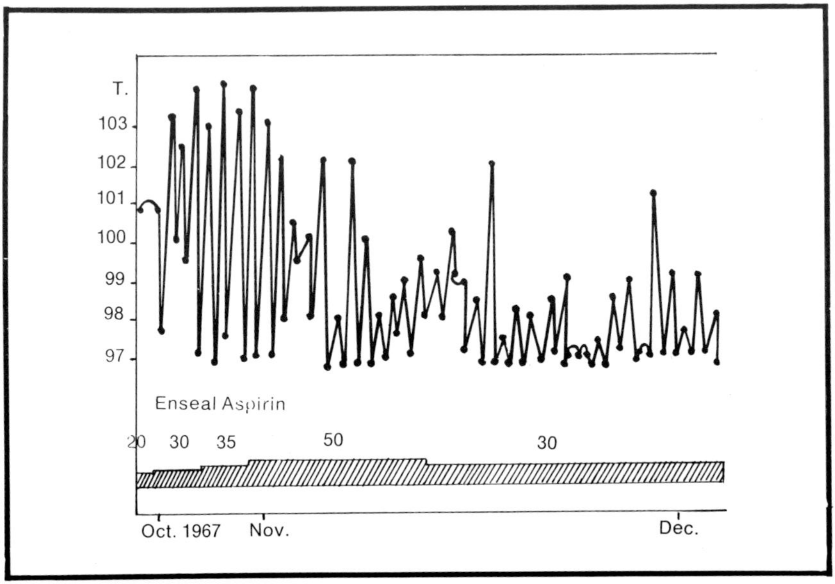
T.
103
102
101
100
99
98
97
Enseal Aspirin
20
30
35
50
30
Oct. 1967
Nov.
Dec.

86

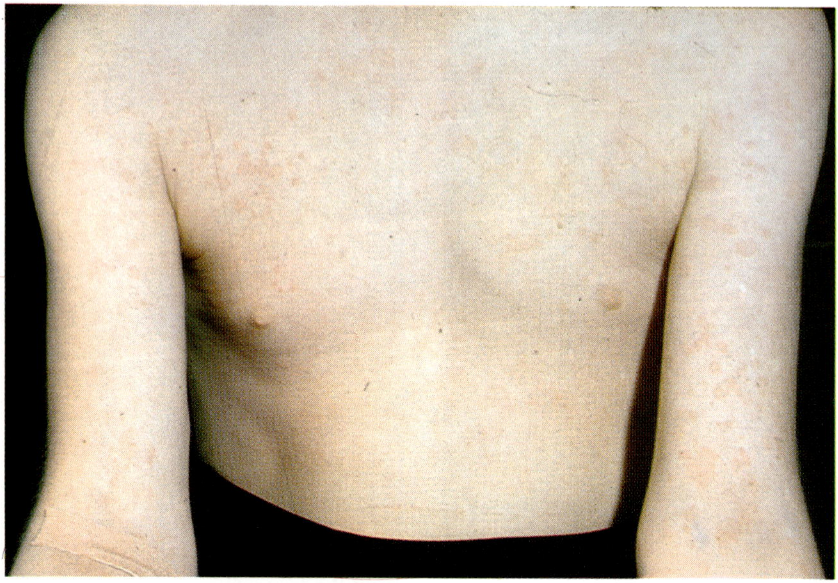

87

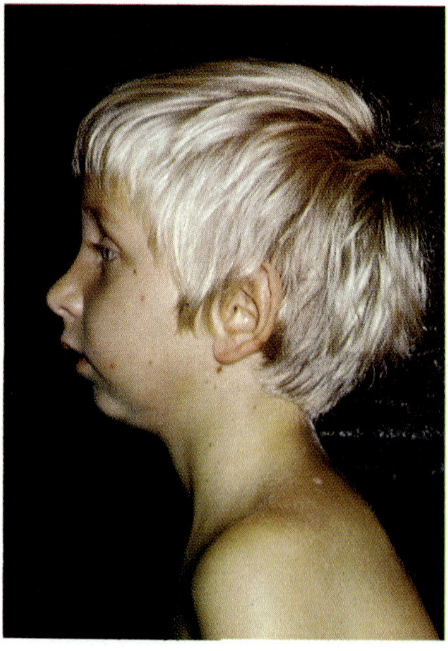

86 Macular rash involving the face arms and legs, and sometimes the trunk accompanies the fever in about 50% o cases.

87 Micrognathia-under-development of the jaw may be associated with involvement of the temporomandibula joints.

88

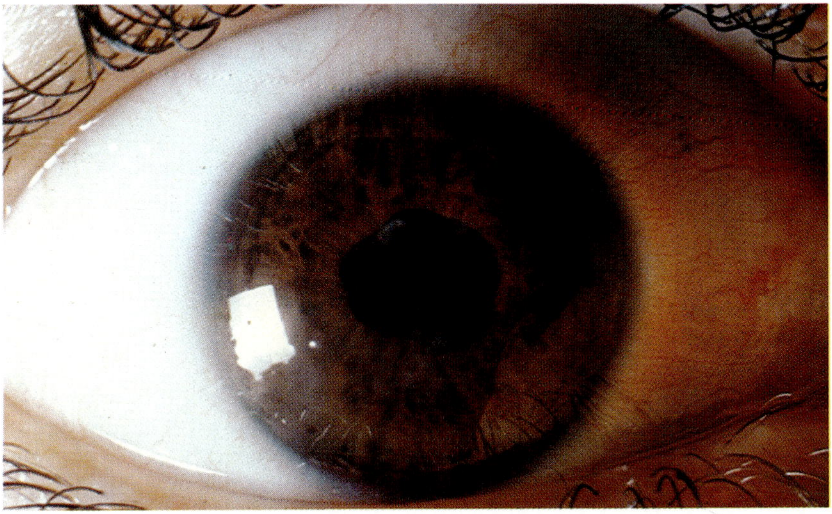

88 Iridocyclitis in Still's disease. The incidence is higher in patients with pauci-articular disease, in girls, and in those with positive antinuclear antibodies.

89

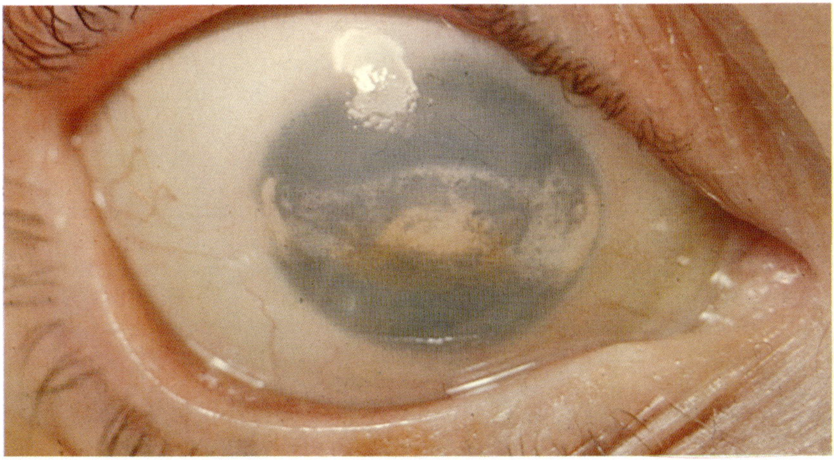

89 Band keratopathy resulting from severe iridocyclitis.

3 Seronegative spondarthritides

This title is used to describe a number of diseases (psoriatic arthritis, Reiter's syndrome, ankylosing spondylitis, enteropathic arthritis and Behçet's disease) which, although originally considered to be variants of rheumatoid arthritis, exhibit certain important differences. In particular, as the name implies, all show a negative test for rheumatoid factor, and in each there is a tendency to involvement of the sacro-iliac joints in the inflammatory process. In addition there are other overlapping features including the occurrence of uveitis, absence of subcutaneous nodules, the similarity of the skin and nail changes in psoriatic arthritis and Reiter's syndrome, and the occasional occurrence of aortitis in ankylosing spondylitis and Reiter's syndrome. Finally, in all of them there is an increased incidence of histo-compatibility antigen HLA–B27 compared with the incidence in the normal population of 8%.

Psoriatic arthritis Psoriasis is a common skin disease, often hereditary, and affecting up to 2% of the population. About 8% of those suffering psoriasis develop an arthritis which differs from rheumatoid arthritis in a number of ways:

1 There is no female preponderance.
2 Rheumatoid factor and subcutaneous nodules are absent.
3 Joint involvement tends to be asymmetrical and may affect the terminal interphalangeal joints and sacro-iliac joints.
4 Skin and joint lesions tend to remit and relapse synchronously.
5 HLA–B27 is found in about 18% of patients with only peripheral joint involvement; if the sacro-iliac joints are involved, this rises to 35%.
6 Systemic complications are rare, but uveitis may occur.

Reiter's syndrome The disease is almost confined to males and is usually sexually transmitted, but may follow epidemic dysentery. A family history of psoriasis is more common in those suffering the disease than in the normal population. The classical triad of urethritis, arthritis, and conjunctivitis is not always complete, conjunctivitis occurring in only 60% of cases. The following are its main features:

1 Genito-urinary involvement: non-specific urethritis, prostatitis, or haemorrhagic cystitis.

2 An inflammatory arthritis predominantly involving the weight-bearing joints (toes, ankles or knees), and often followed by sacro-iliitis with para-spinal ligamentous calcification or ossification.

3 Ocular lesions: conjunctivitis in the early stage, iritis later affecting 10% of patients.

4 Mucosal lesions: shallow penile ulceration, circinate balanitis, and ulceration of the buccal mucosa and tongue.

5 Skin and nail lesions: keratodermia blennorrhagica which may be indistinguishable histologically from pustular psoriasis, and nail dystrophy also closely resembling that seen in psoriasis.

6 Cardiac involvement: rarely aortitis or pericarditis.

7 HLA–B27 is positive in about 75% of cases.

Ankylosing spondylitis Heredity appears to play some part in the aetiology of ankylosing spondylitis, the disease appearing 30 times more commonly in relatives of sufferers than in non-spondylitic controls. Its main features are:

1 A marked male predominance with onset in the late 'teens or early twenties.

2 Bilateral sacro-iliitis usually proceeding to para-spinal ligamentous calcification or ossification with ankylosis of the spinal facet joints.

3 Peripheral joint involvement more common in the hips and shoulders than elsewhere.

4 A high incidence (about 25%) of iritis.

5 Rarely aortitis or pulmonary fibrosis affecting the upper lung fields.

6 In this disease HLA–B27 is positive in about 95% of patients.

Enteropathic arthritis Arthritis may complicate ulcerative colitis, Crohn's disease (regional ileitis), or Whipple's disease. For practical purposes the forms of arthritis which occur in ulcerative colitis and Crohn's disease are similar and may be considered together. There appear to be two quite distinct entities:

1 A peripheral arthritis occurring in between 10–20% of patients, and with a close temporal relation to the activity of the bowel disease. Lower limb joints, particularly knees and ankles, are involved more commonly than others, and the arthritis tends to be transitory and to flit from joint to joint. Cure of the bowel disease leads to remission of the arthritis.

2 Sacro-iliitis which may proceed to spinal ligamentous calcification or ossification, giving a clinical and radiological picture indistinguishable from ankylosing spondylitis. Unlike the peripheral arthritis there is no temporal relation to the bowel disease, nor does treatment of the latter affect the course of the spondylitis.

3 In the presence of sacro-iliitis HLA–B27 positivity amounts to about 67%, but if peripheral arthritis occurs alone, positivity is no more than in the normal population.

Behçet's disease This is a rare condition, first described in 1908 as a triad of relapsing iritis, genital and oral ulceration, and arthritis. Other features include vasculitis, particularly a tendency to venous thrombosis, and neurological defects. As in other members of the group sacro-iliitis may occur in addition to peripheral arthritis, and there is an increased incidence (albeit small) of HLA–B27.

Psoriatic arthritis

Psoriatic arthritis should be suspected in patients with an asymetrical large joint arthritis, who are seronegative, and in particular if there is a family history of psoriasis, since the arthritis may sometimes precede the skin lesions by months or even years.

90

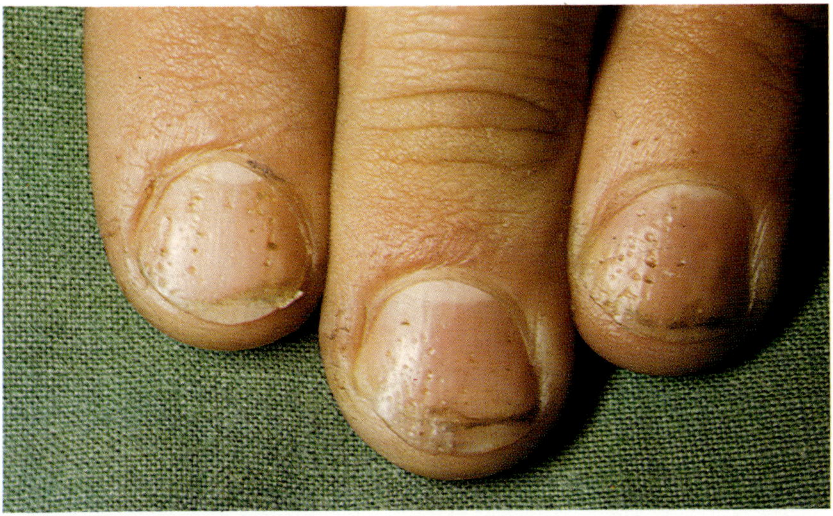

90 Early psoriasis of the nails ('thimble pitting'). *(Picture by kind permission of Dr GM Levene, St John's Hospital, London)*

91 Advanced nail psoriasis shows dystrophy of the nails, discolouration and sub-ungual separation. Note the swelling of several terminal interphalangeal joints associated with the neighbouring nail dystrophy.

It would seem that nail involvement in some way enhances liability to develop arthropathy, since 80% of patients with psoriatic arthritis have both skin and nail lesions.

92 Early psoriatic arthritis showing nail changes and redness and swelling of several terminal interphalangeal joints.

93 Early psoriatic arthritis. Close-up view of same patient (**92**).

91

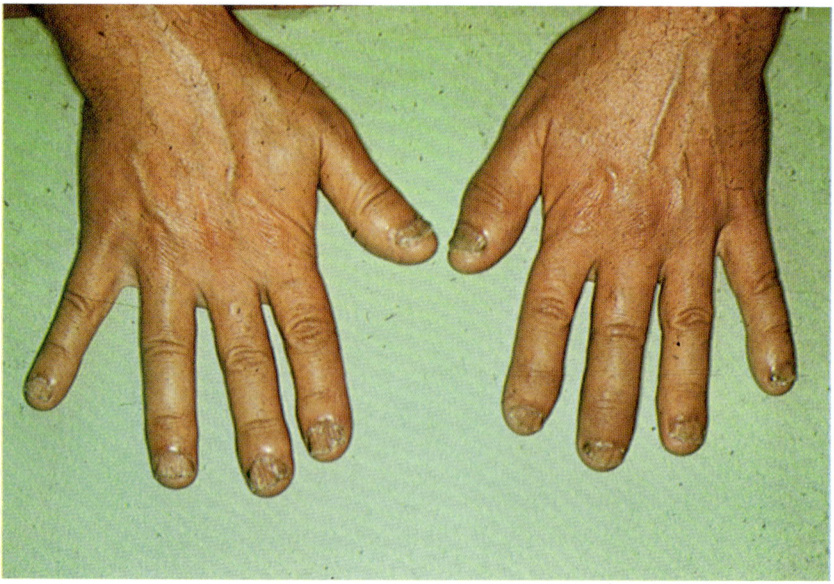

92

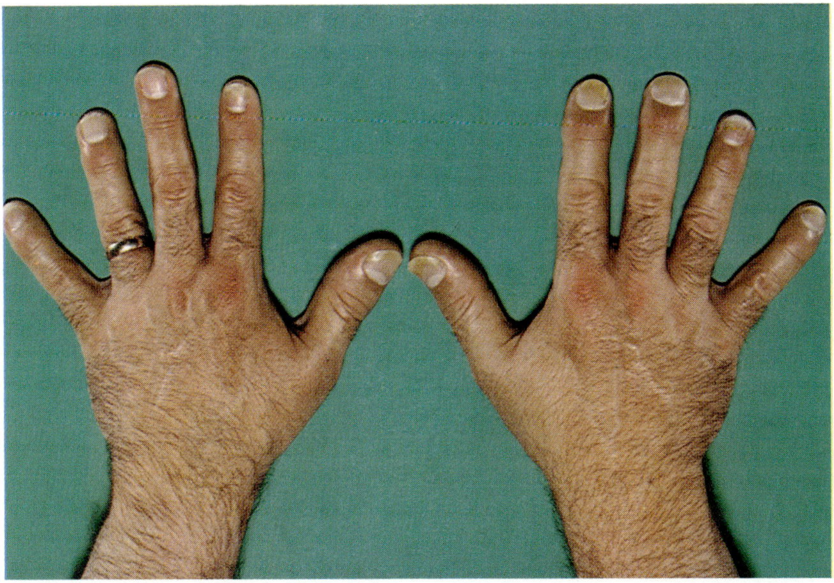

93

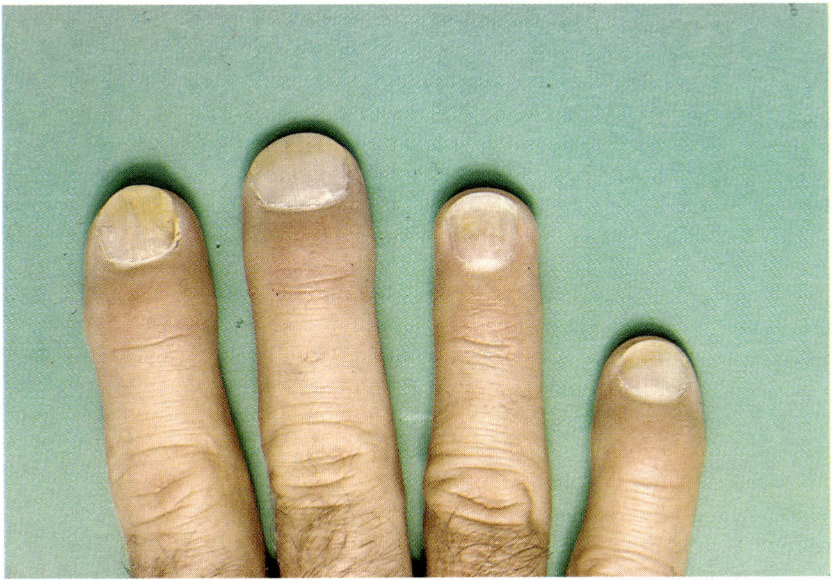

94

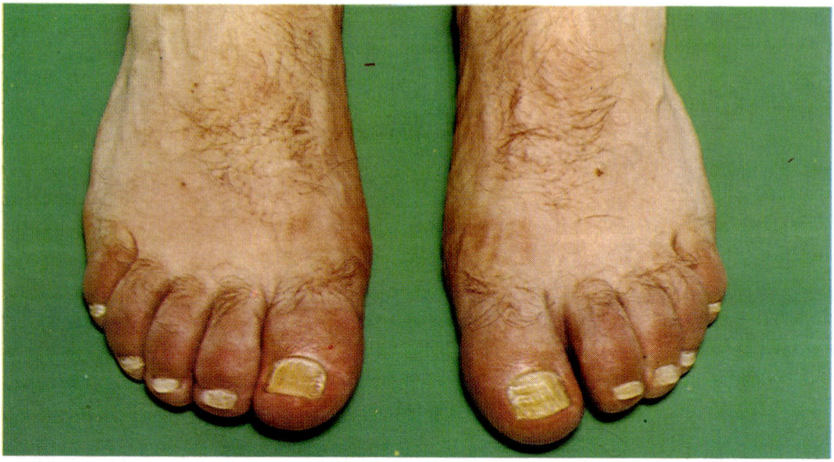

94 Psoriatic arthritis of the feet. Again there are nail changes and involvement of the terminal joints of the toes.

95

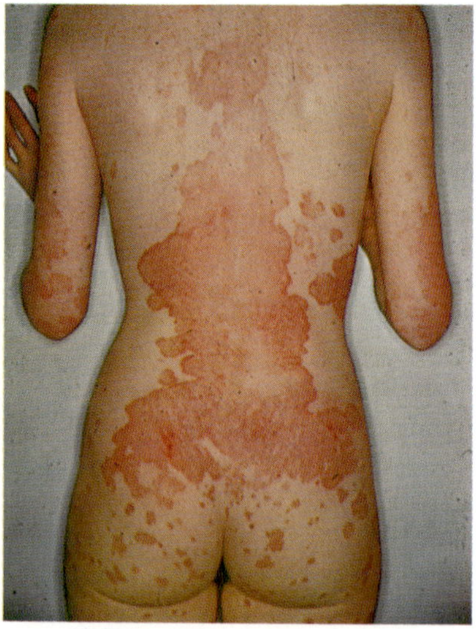

95 Typical psoriasis involving the trunk.

96

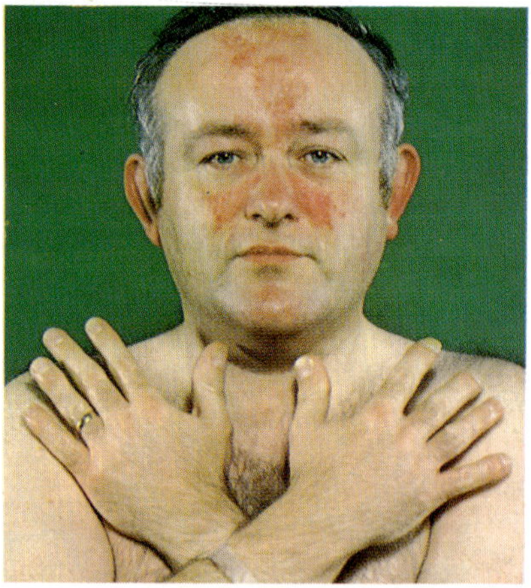

96 Psoriasis affecting the face, with nail dystrophy and terminal interphalangeal arthritis.

97

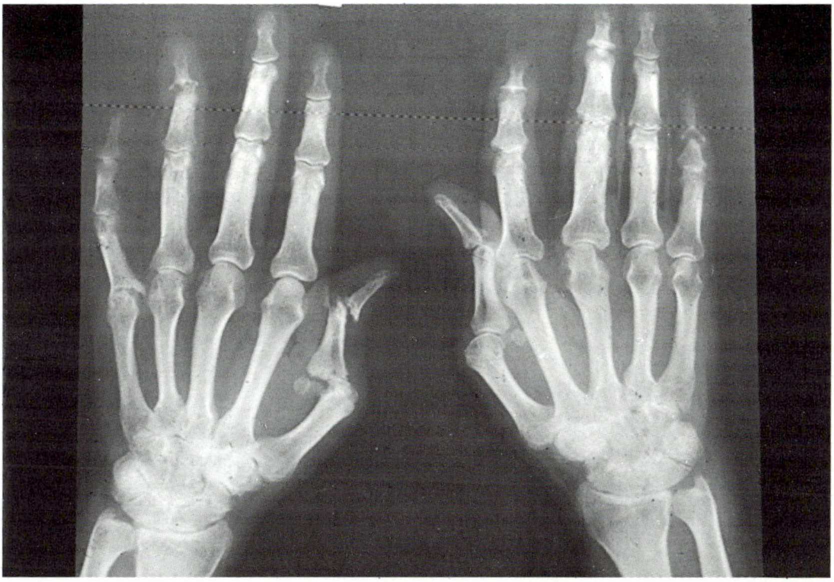

97 **Early psoriatic arthritis.** Note erosive changes in the left ring and right little finger terminal interphalangeal joints. Cartilage loss and erosions in other joints resemble changes seen in rheumatoid arthritis.

98

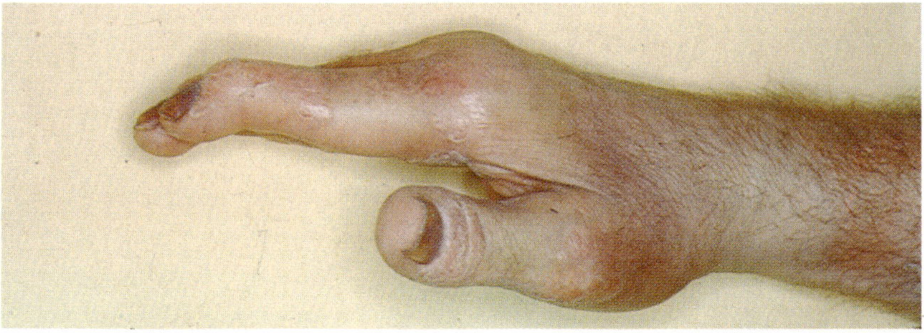

98 **Psoriatic arthritis** involving nails and distal interphalangeal joints.

99

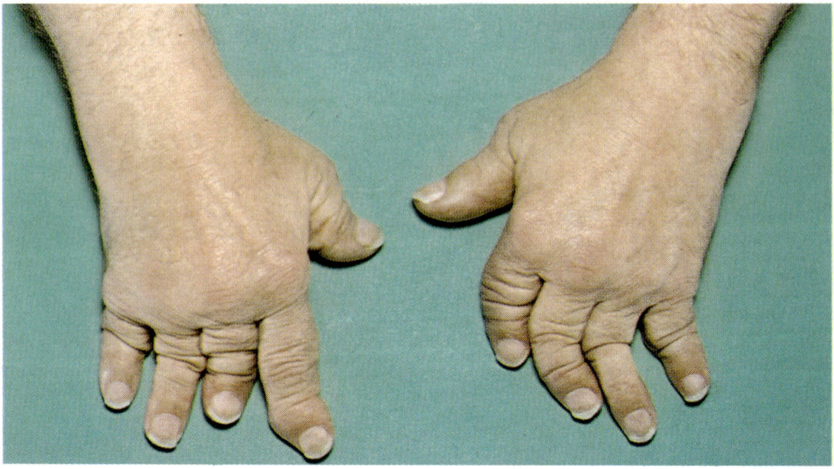

99 Advanced psoriatic arthritis. Although often benign and only slowly progressive, this form of arthritis can sometimes be extremely destructive, resulting in absorption of phalanges, giving rise to the 'main-en-lorgnette' phenomenon as seen here.

100 Lateral view of the same hands (**99**).

100

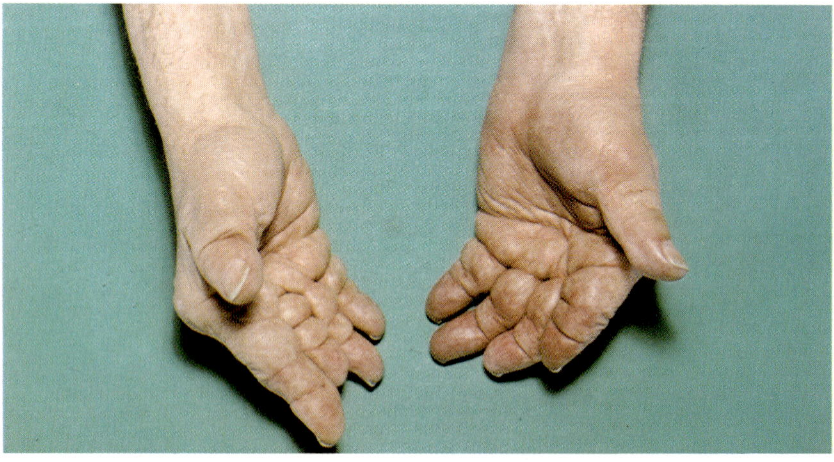

101

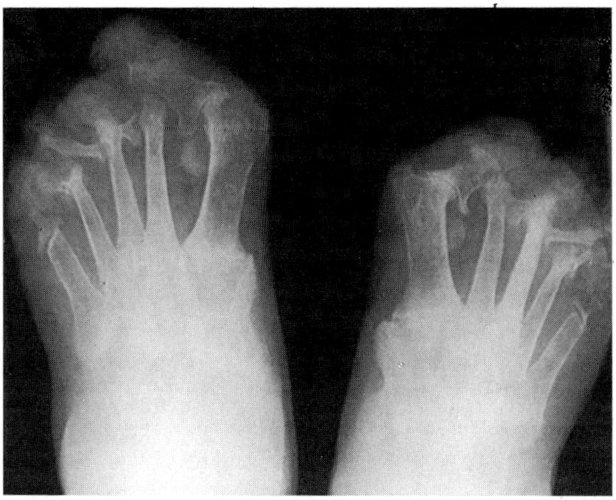

101 Advanced psoriatic arthritis showing severe destructive changes.

102

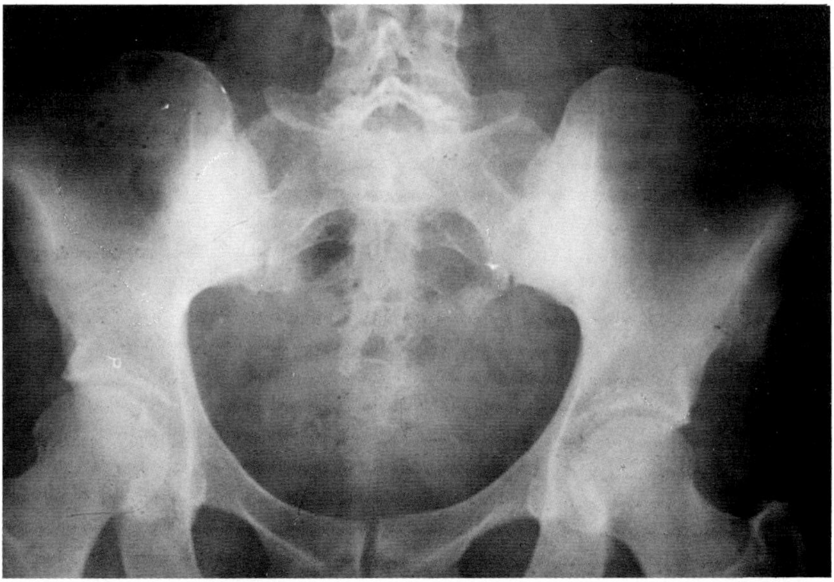

102 Bilateral sacro-iliitis occurs in 10–30% of patients with psoriasis, sometimes followed by para-spinal ligamentous calcification or ossification closely resembling ankylosing spondylitis (so called psoriasis spondylitica).

Reiter's syndrome

The classical triad in this disease is non-specific urethritis, arthritis, and conjunctivitis. Arthritis usually follows the urethritis after an interval of 1–3 weeks, and in the early stages is nearly always confined to the joints of the lower limb, particularly the small joints of the toes and ankles. The urethritis may be transient and overlooked by the physician, or concealed by the patient, who may be too worried or ashamed to reveal it. Prostatitis should be looked for, and the secretion examined after prostatic massage. In the same way, the conjunctivitis may be so transient as to be forgotten by the patient. However, suspicion of the diagnosis should be aroused if the patient is a young male with an acute mono- or polyarthritis affecting the feet, ankles or knees.

103 Acute non-specific urethritis. Meatitis and circinate balanitis may follow.

104 Circinate balanatis.

105 Conjunctivitis is not an essential part of the triad of Reiter's syndrome, as it may be absent in 40% of cases. It is always bilateral, and may be transient and missed by the clinician.

103

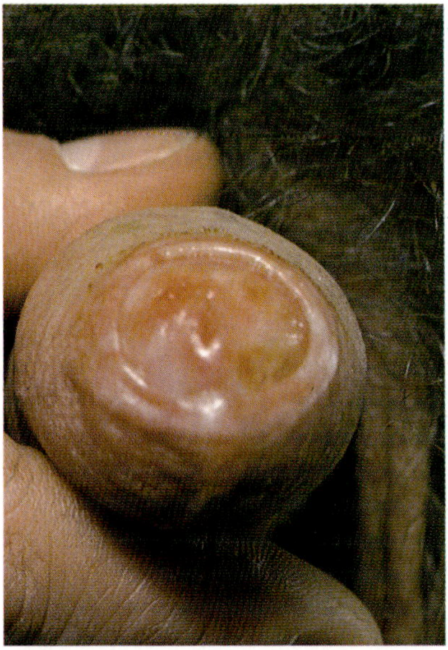

104

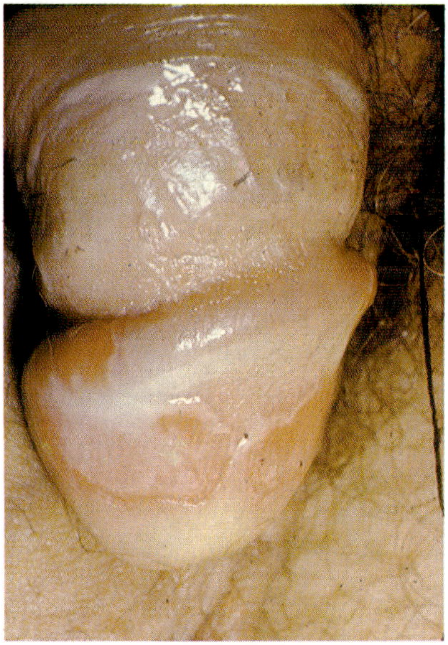

105

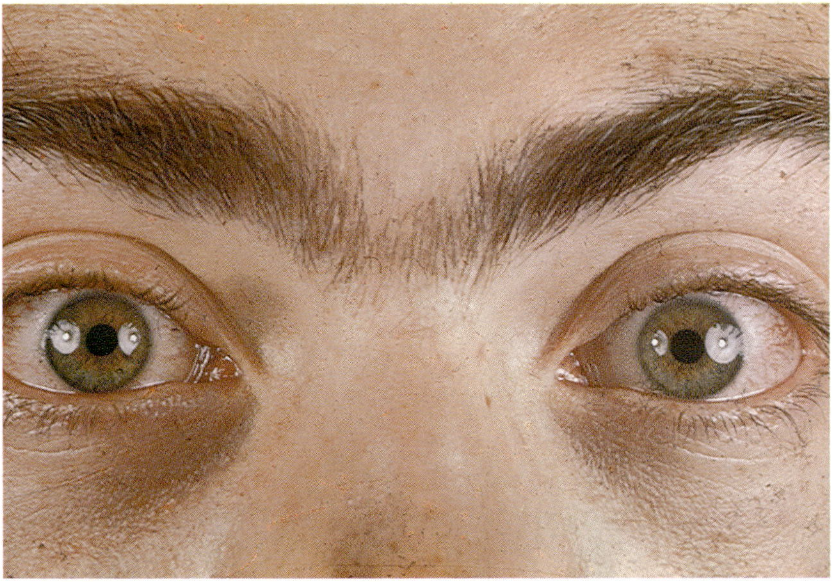

106 Acute Reiter's syndrome. There is marked swelling and redness of the small joints of the toes of the left foot and destructive changes have shortened the great toe. Note the similarity of the skin lesions (keratodermia blennorrhagica) to pustular psoriasis and of the nail lesions to those of advanced psoriasis. In Reiter's syndrome the nails are sometimes completely shed.

107 Periostitis over the lower end of both medial malleoli. X-ray changes may show osteoporosis around affected joints, which may later proceed to erosion and destructive changes as seen in other inflammatory arthritides. Periostitis around infected joints is typical.

108 Sacro-iliitis may occur, followed by para-spinal ligamentous calcification or ossification with a final picture closely resembling ankylosing spondylitis. Note sclerosis and erosions affecting the lower pole of both sacro-iliac joints.

106

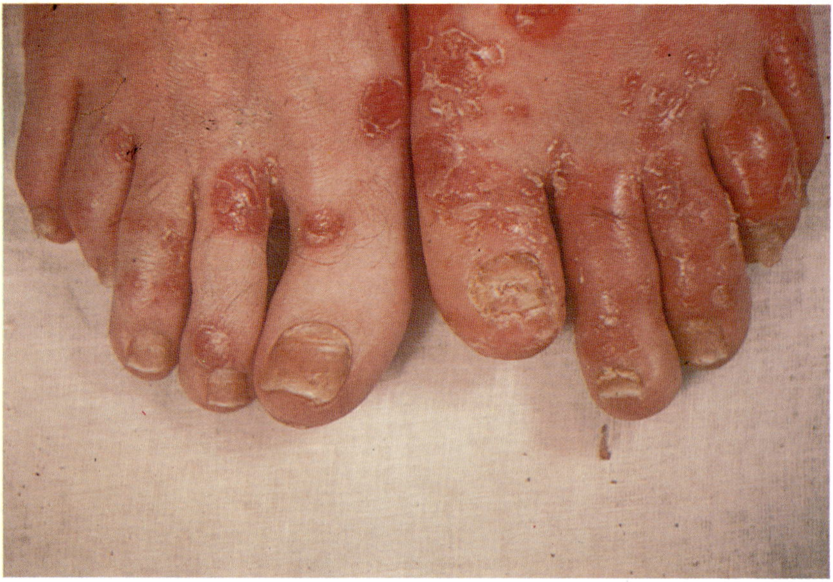

107

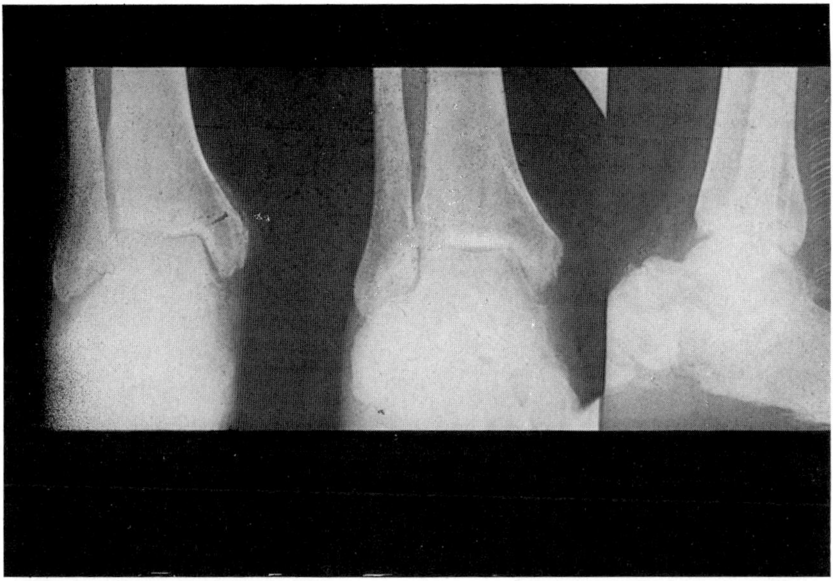

108

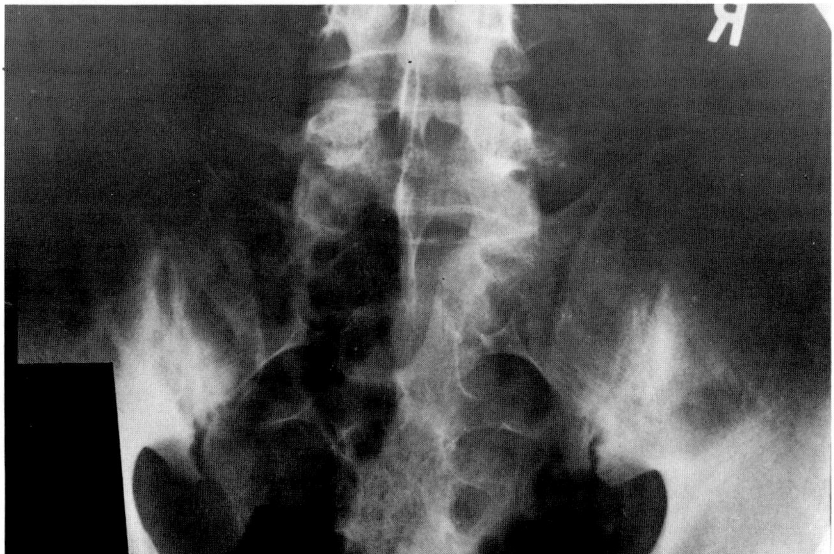

109 Painful heel is a common symptom. X-ray may show calcaneal spurring and sometimes erosion of the os calcis.

110 Keratodermia blennorrhagica occurs in more severe relapsing cases, and is often confined to the feet and lower legs. Both clinically and histologically, these skin lesions closely resemble pustular psoriasis. Involvement of the soles of the feet is typical.

111 Advanced keratodermia blennorrhagica of the feet and lower legs.

112 Nail dystrophy in Reiter's syndrome with inflammatory changes in the distal interphalangeal joints of the toes.

109

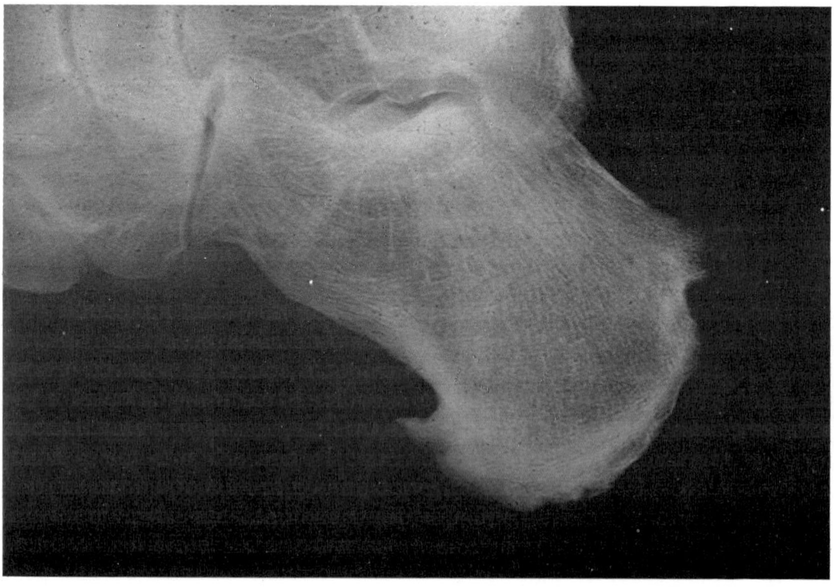

110

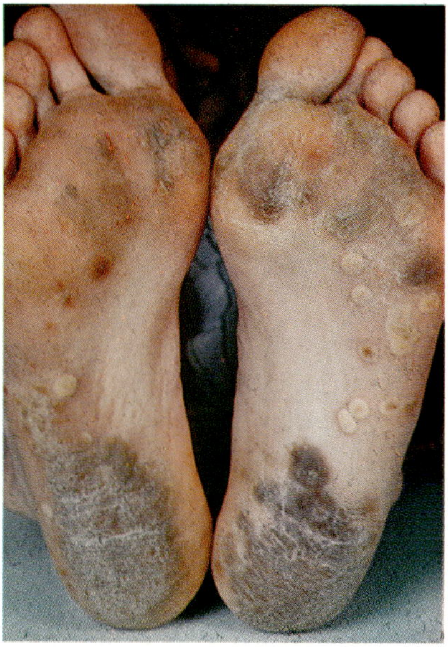

111

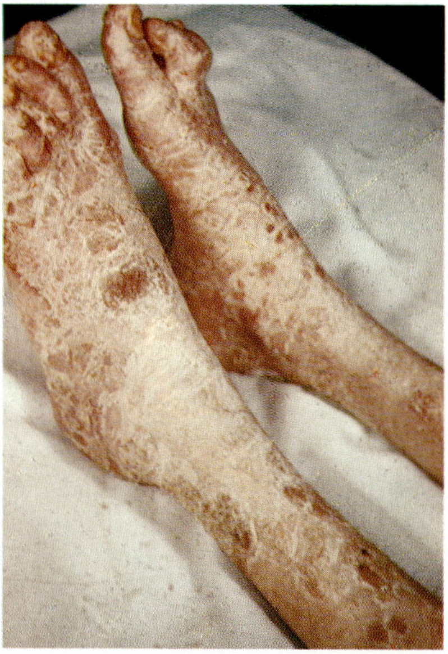

112

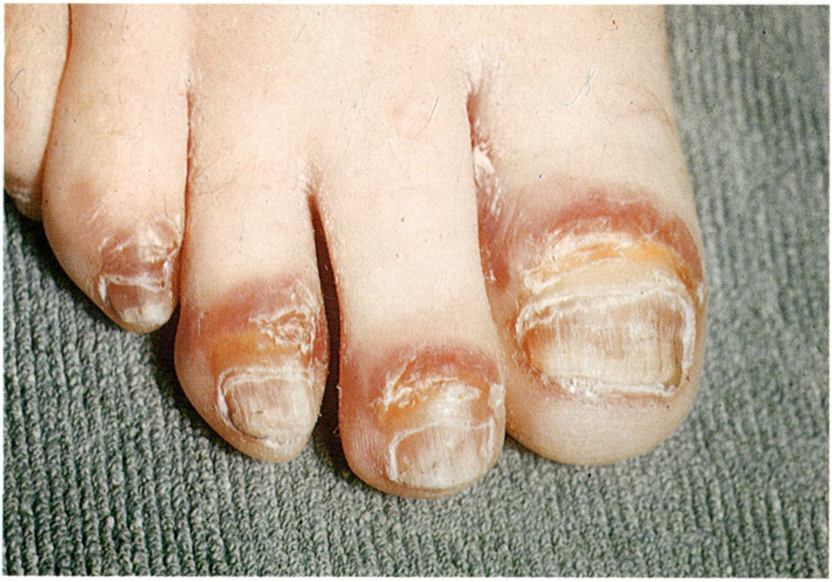

113 Balanitis of the penis. Superficial ulceration of mucous membranes occurs in the more severe type of case. Similar changes may affect the buccal mucosa. Ulcers around the penile meatus are also characteristic.

114 Acute iritis, often recurrent, affects about 20% of patients with Reiter's syndrome and is usually associated with severe and relapsing disease. Note that unlike conjunctivitis, iritis is almost always unilateral.

115 Acute iritis. Close-up view of the same patient (**114**).

113

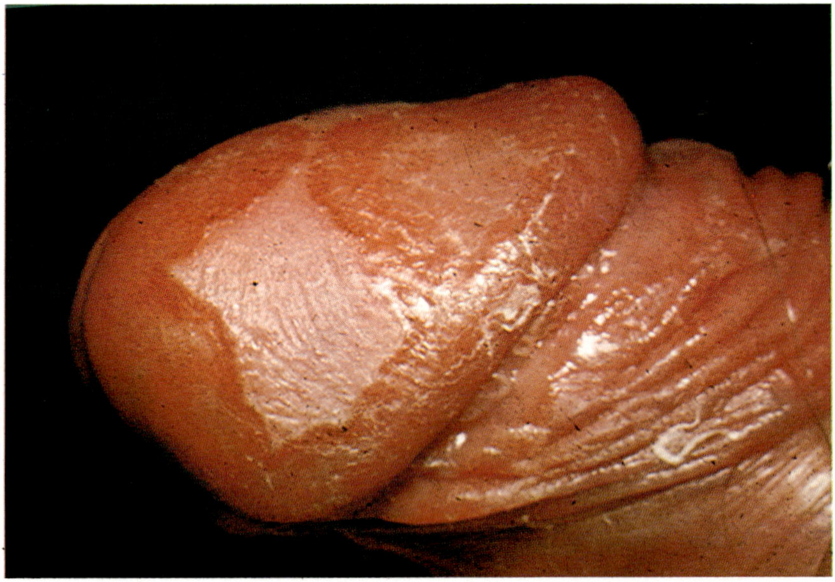

114

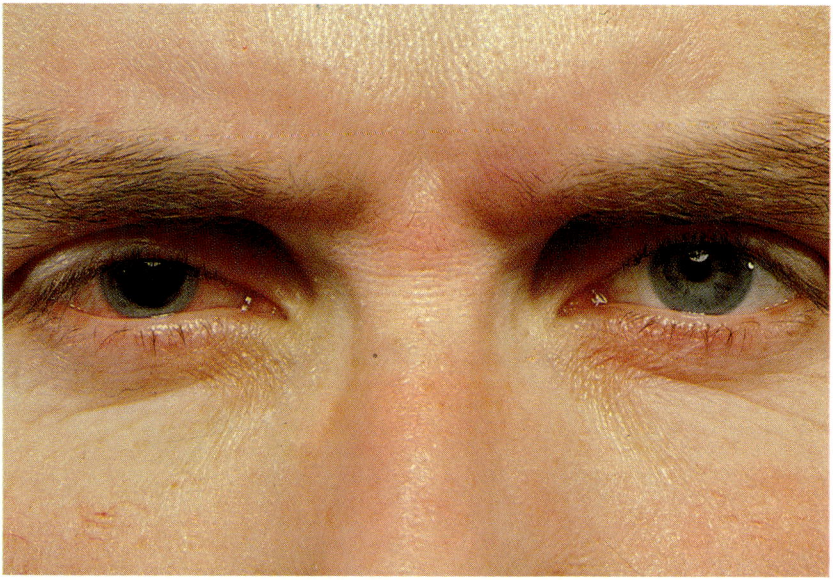

115

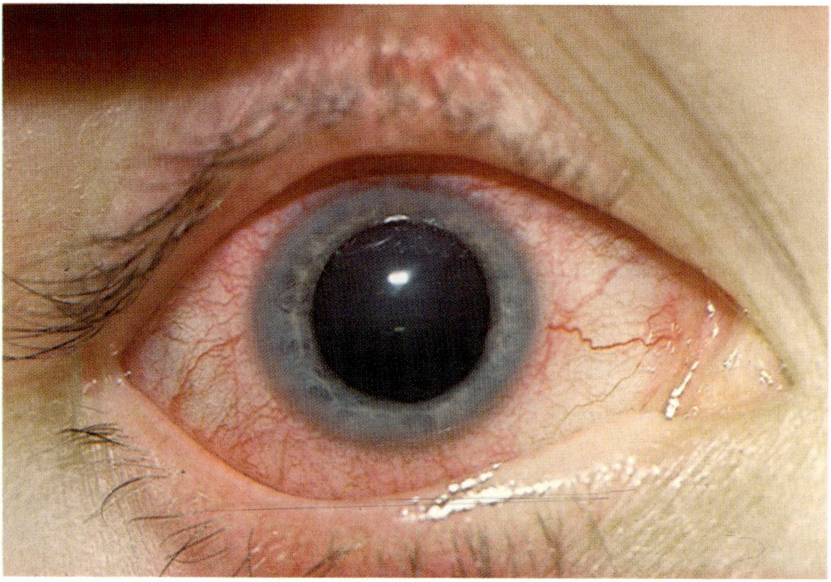

Ankylosing spondylitis

This disease is much more common in men than in women (ratio 8:1), and symptoms are usually first apparent in the late teens or early twenties, with increasing aching and early morning stiffness in the lower back. Many cases remain mild and only slowly progressive while others exhibit a progressive advance of the disease up the spine, with consequent spinal ligamentous calcification and ossification which may result in total rigidity of the entire spinal column. Involvement of the hip and shoulder joints is not uncommon, but other peripheral joints are rarely involved. Nodules are absent, tests for rheumatoid factor generally negative, but at least 95% of patients are HLA–B27 positive.

116 Typical kyphosis where the disease has progressed to involve the dorsal spine.

117 Typical kyphosis. Posterior view of the same patient (**116**).

118 Forward flexion is achieved by movement of the hip joints. The lumbar and dorsal spines are totally stiff.

119 Limitation of side flexion is an early sign and will often distinguish the disease from mechanical derangements of the spine, in which side flexion is remarkably free and painless.

116

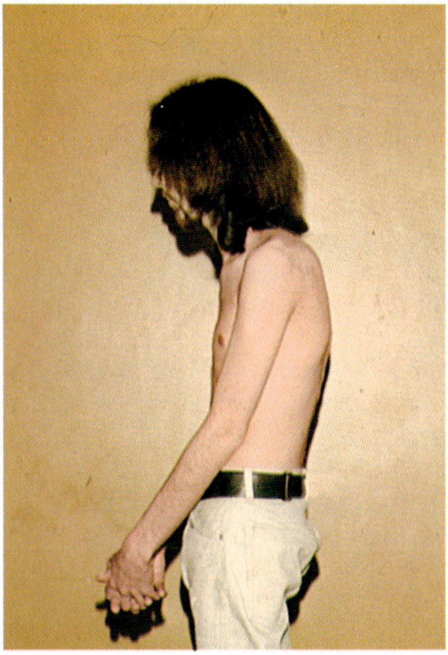

117

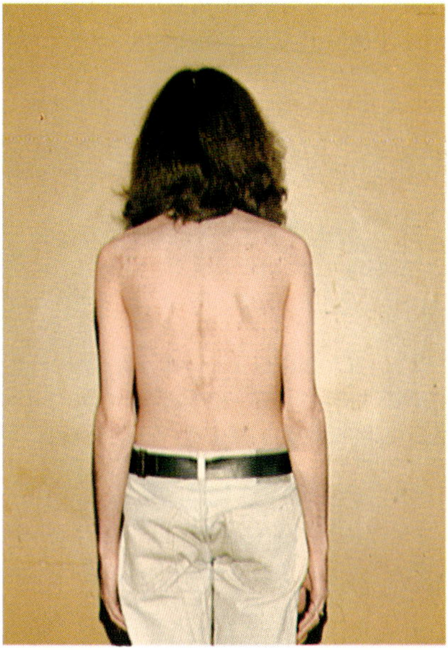

118

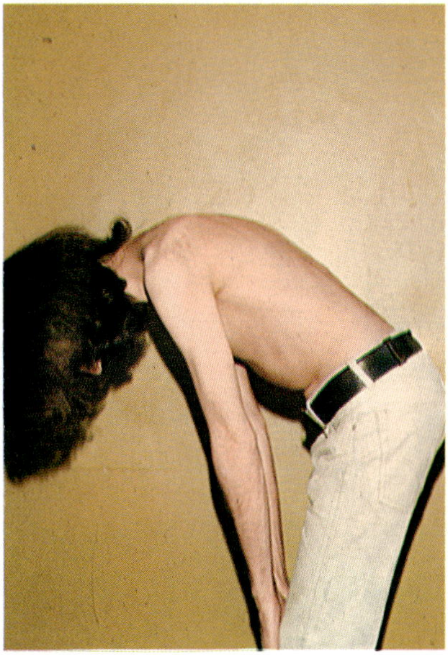

119

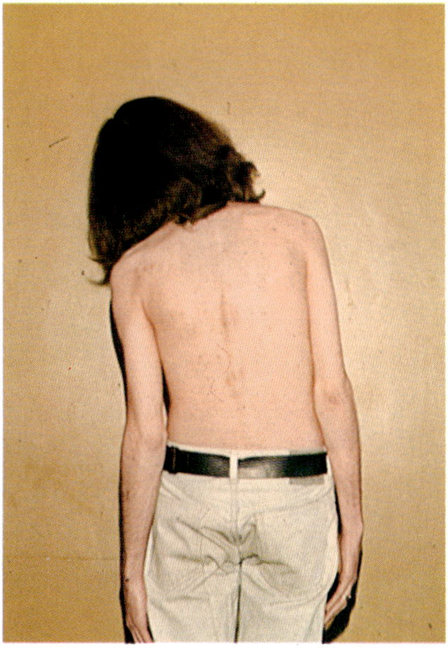

120 Sacro-iliac joints. Radiograph shows erosion and sclerosis of the margins of the joint (as seen in the right joint), proceeding to ankylosis (as seen in the lower pole of the left joint). Note also erosion of the symphysis pubis. A fluffy periosteal reaction is often also seen at the site of muscle attachments, particularly around the iliac crests and lower pubic rami.

121 Ankylosing spondylitis: late X-ray changes. The sacro-iliac joints are now obliterated by ankylosis, and ossification has occurred in the paraspinal ligaments. Note also affection of the hip joints.

122 Calcification of the lateral spinal ligaments: revealed by anteroposterior view of the lumbar spine. The earliest change of this type is typically seen at the dorso-lumbar junction.

123 Patchy calcification of the anterior spinal ligament revealed by lateral X-rays of the lumbar spine.

120

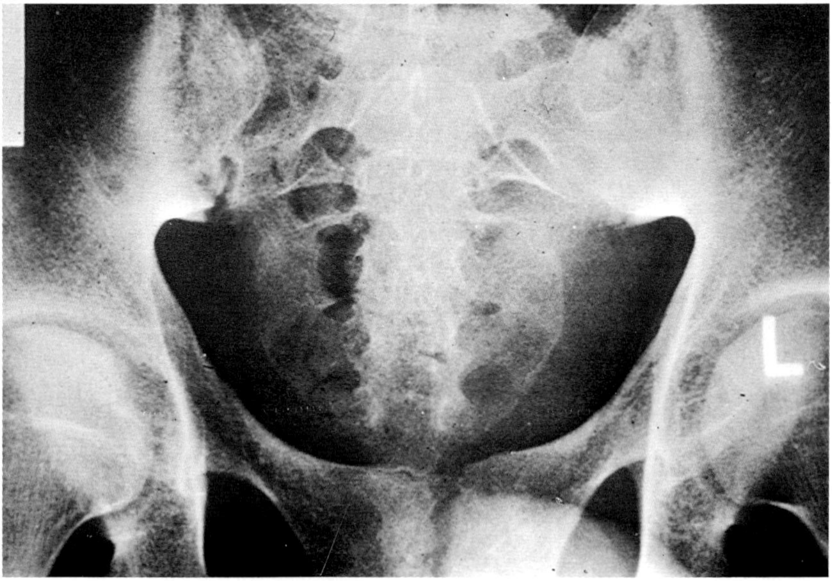

121

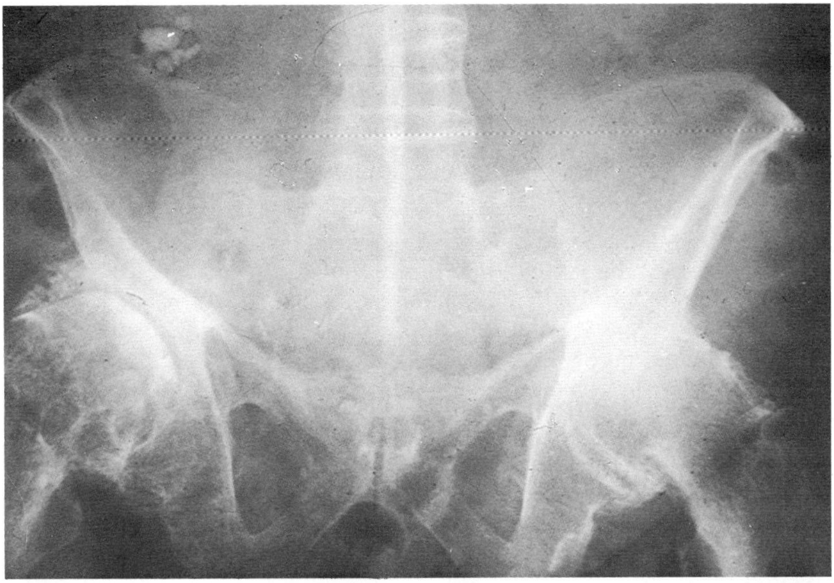

122

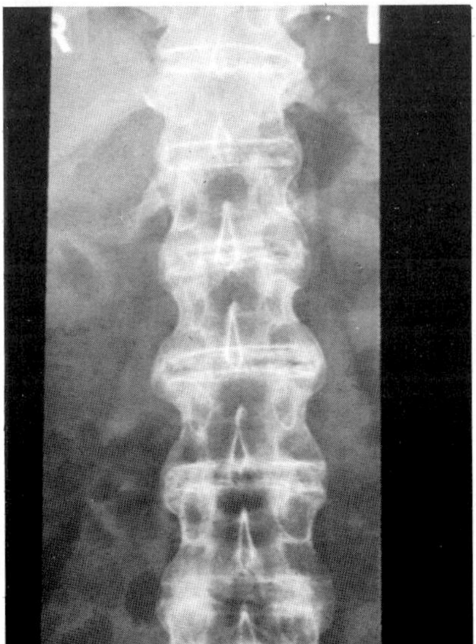

123

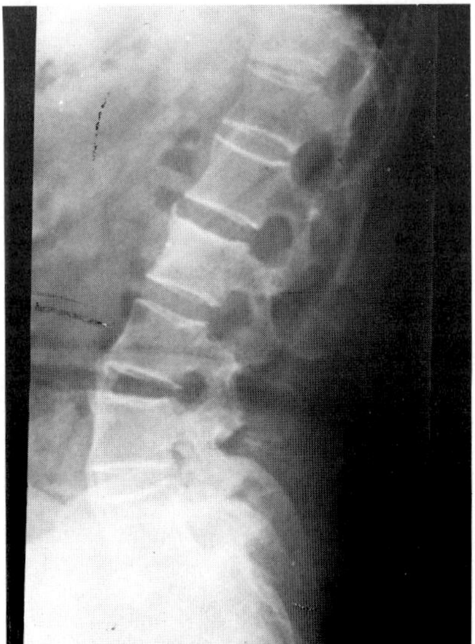

124 The cervical spine in ankylosing spondylitis, with calcification of the anterior spinal ligament. Atlanto-axial subluxation may occur as it does in rheumatoid arthritis (see page 127), but subluxation at lower levels rarely if ever occurs, presumably because the vertebrae are splinted by the calcified ligaments. Due to its rigidity however, the cervical spine is unduly susceptible to trauma, and fracture may occur following relatively trivial injury.

125 Erosion of the manubriosternal joint may occur giving rise to local tenderness and pain in deep breathing.

126 The so-called 'Romanus lesion', or anterior spondylitis. These are probably inflammatory lesions involving the adjacent anterior parts of vertebral bodies, which often heal spontaneously and are usually symptomless.

124

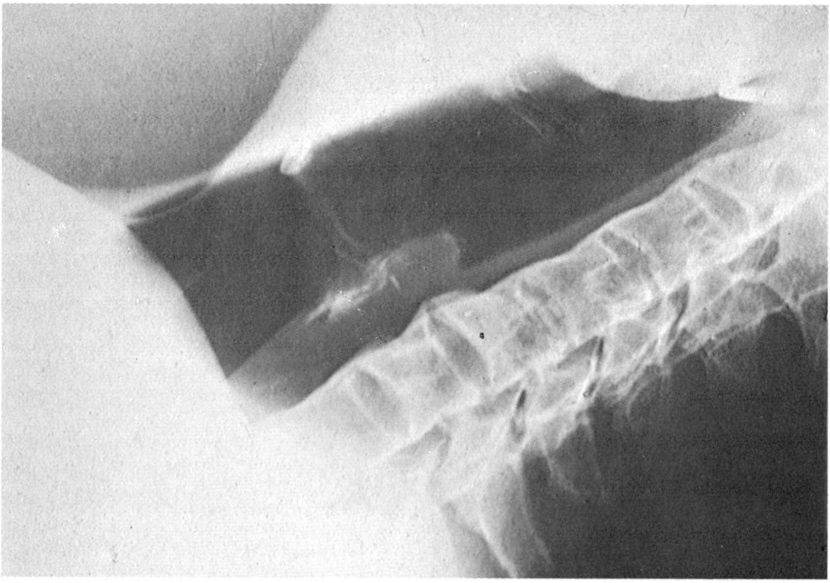

125

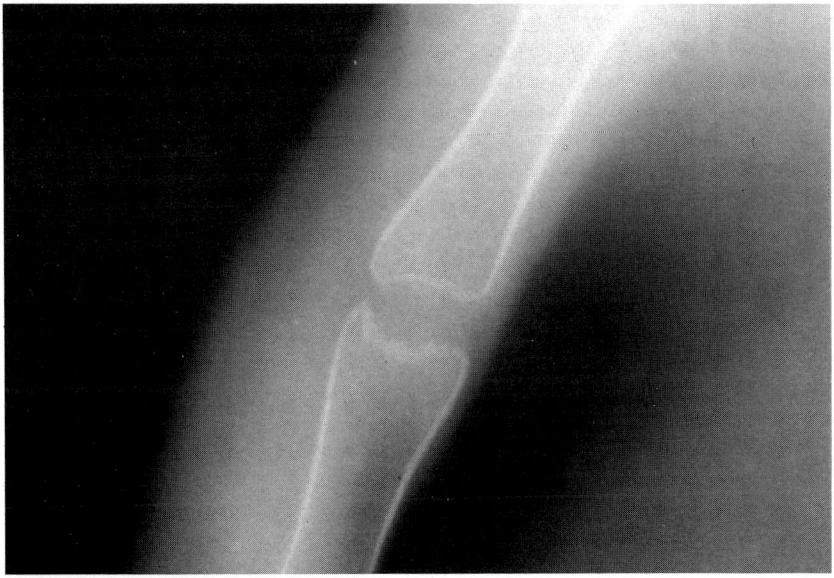

126

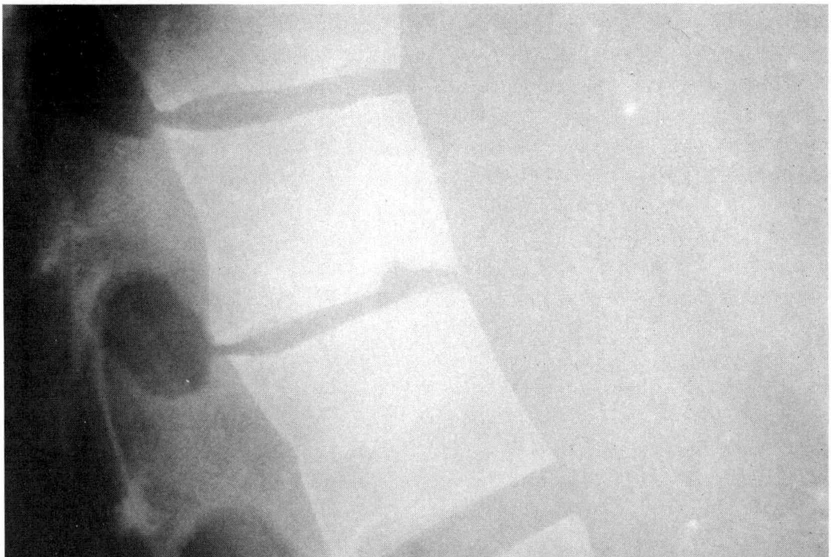

127 **Iritis** is the commonest complication of ankylosing spondylitis and occurs in about 25% of patients. Recurrent attacks may occur over a period of years. This illustration of acute iritis shows also a hypopyon.

128 **Posterior synechiae** with permanent damage to vision may develop as a result of repeated attacks of iritis.

129 **Chronic iritis.**

127

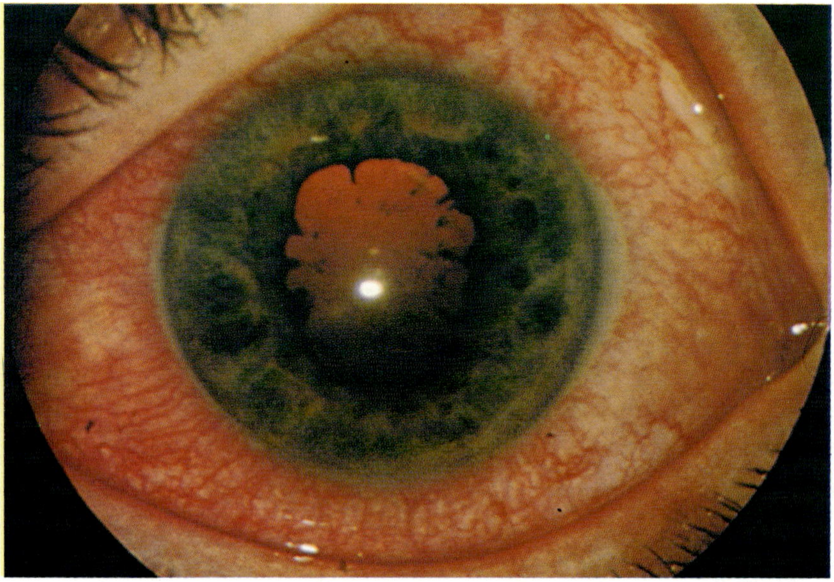

128

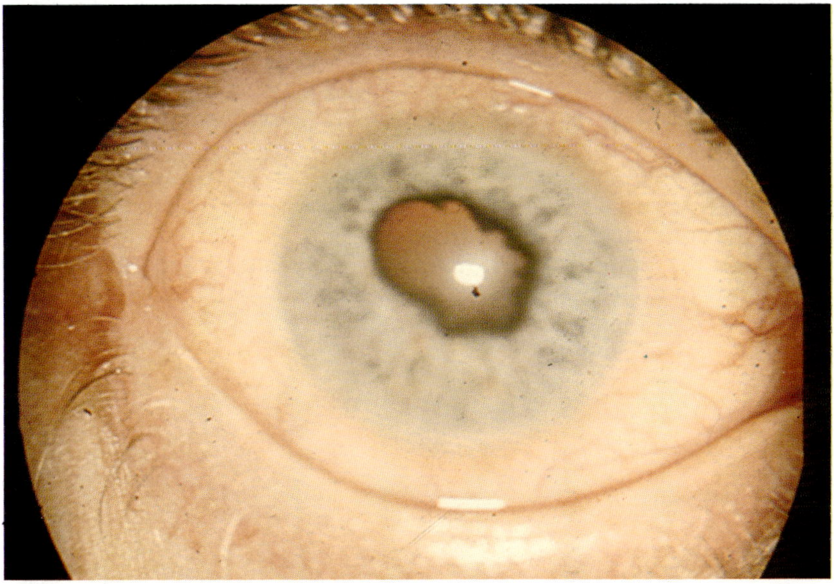

129

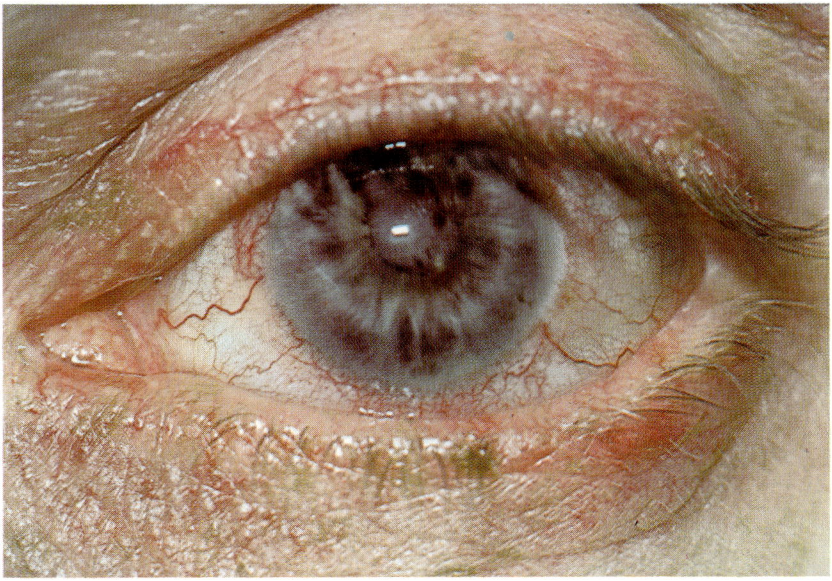

Enteropathic arthritis

This may present as a complication of ulcerative colitis, Crohn's disease (regional ileitis), or Whipple's disease. All these bowel diseases may be associated with sacro-iliitis and para-spinal ligamentous calcification. A peripheral arthritis may also occur, usually predominantly affecting the joints of the lower limb.

130 Ulcerative colitis and effusion into both knees. The latter cleared up when the colitis was successfully treated.

Unlike the peripheral arthritis, sacro-iliitis and spondylitis bear no temporal relationship to the bowel disease, nor is their course affected by successful treatment of the bowel.

130

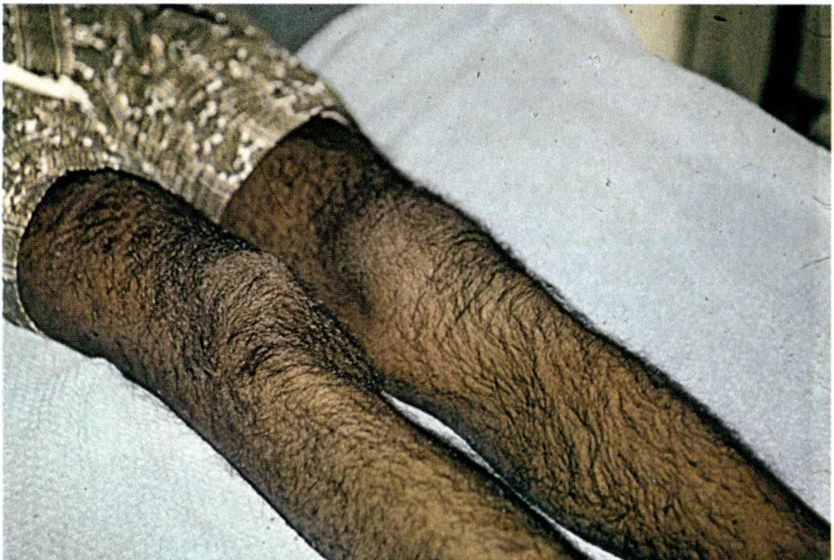

Behçet's disease

131 Genital ulceration is a common feature and often affects the scrotum as shown here.

132 Vasculitis in Behçet's disease causing gangrene of the great and little toes. The patient subsequently underwent an above knee amputation.

133 Arteriogram of the same patient (**132**) showing a popliteal aneurysm.

131

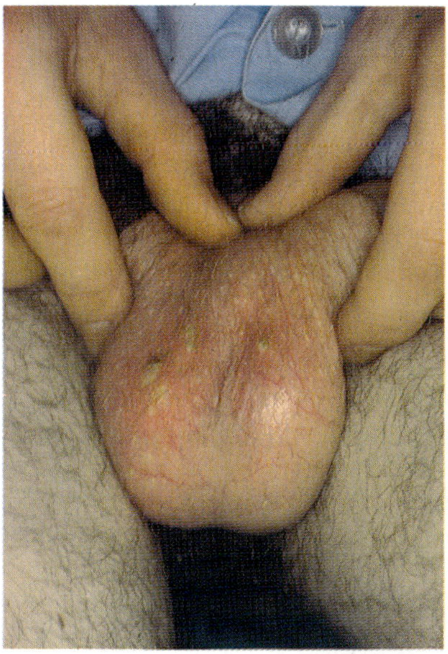

132

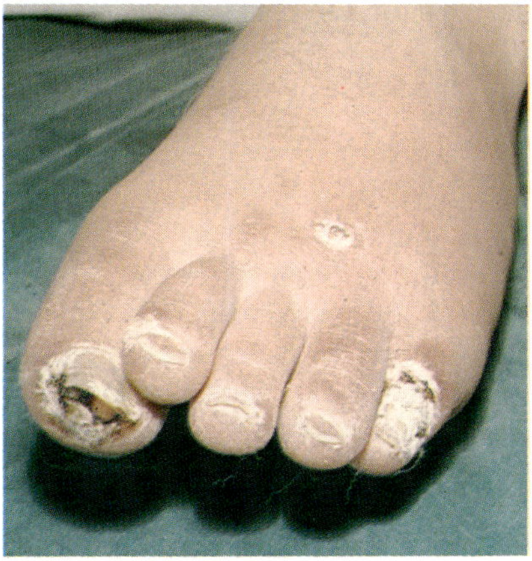

133

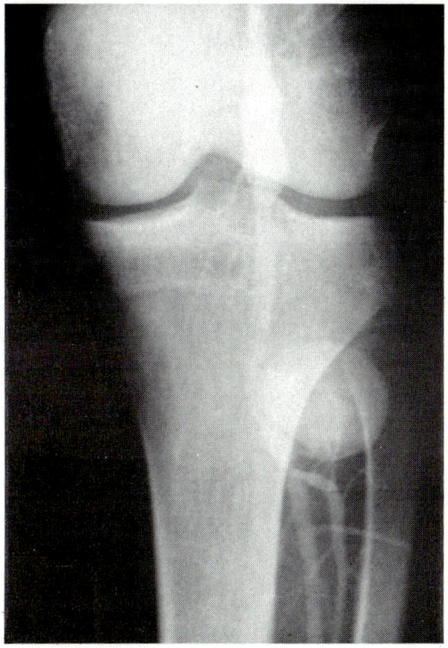

4 Degenerative joint disease

Affection of synovial joints by degenerative processes is now generally known as osteoarthrosis (formerly osteoarthritis). Degeneration of intervertebral discs, which are fibrocartilaginous joints (synchondroses), is known as spondylosis.

Osteoarthrosis Although primarily considered to be part of the ageing process, osteoarthrosis appears to have a number of factors in its aetiology. There is evidence of a genetic determinant, but in addition, occupation, obesity, or previous injury to the joint may determine its site and severity. More recently, the finding of particles of hydroxyapatite in joints affected by degenerative change suggests that there may, in addition, be a biochemical factor.

The major lesion in affected joints is in articular cartilage, which shows softening, fibrillation and flaking. The underlying causes of these changes are still obscure, but it would seem that both mechanical and biochemical factors play a part. Subchondral bone undergoes thickening and sclerosis, and cysts may occur in deeper layers, perhaps due to herniation of synovial fluid through breaks in the trabeculae. Osteophyte formation at the margin of affected joints is characteristic.

In general, osteoarthrosis may be distinguished from rheumatoid arthritis by the absence of signs of inflammation in affected joints and of a disturbance of general health, together with the finding of a normal ESR and negative tests for rheumatoid factor. Radiological changes do not necessarily mirror the symptomatology. Disability is usually not serious unless the hip joints are affected.

Spondylosis Degeneration of intervertebral discs may be accompanied by osteoarthrosis of the diarthrodial (facet) joints. Radiological changes of disc degeneration are almost universal in the older age group but do not necessarily indicate that they are the cause of local pain and stiffness. As with osteoarthrosis of peripheral joints, spondylosis rarely causes major disability, but advanced changes in the cervical region of the spine may result in local compression of the spinal cord giving rise to long tract signs – usually a spastic quadriplegia.

Osteoarthrosis

134 Heberden's nodes (involvement of the terminal interphalangeal joints of the fingers) are the most characteristic feature of osteoarthrosis of the hands. In the earliest stage, swelling over the lateral parts of the joint may have an overlying cystic feel, later becoming hard and bony.

135 Advanced Heberden's nodes affecting all the terminal interphalangeal joints. Lateral deviation of the terminal phalanx may occur as seen in the left index and middle fingers.

134

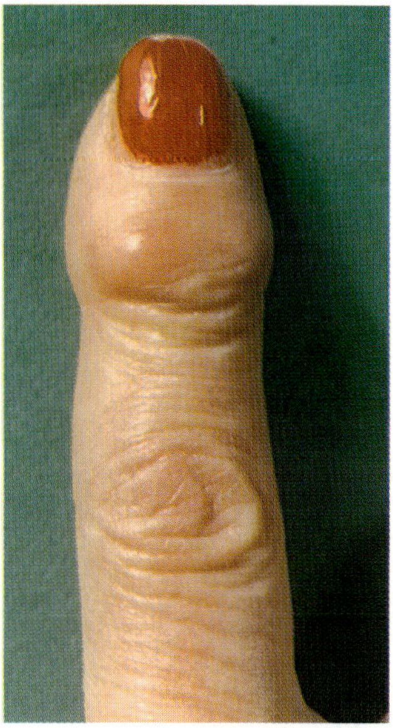

135

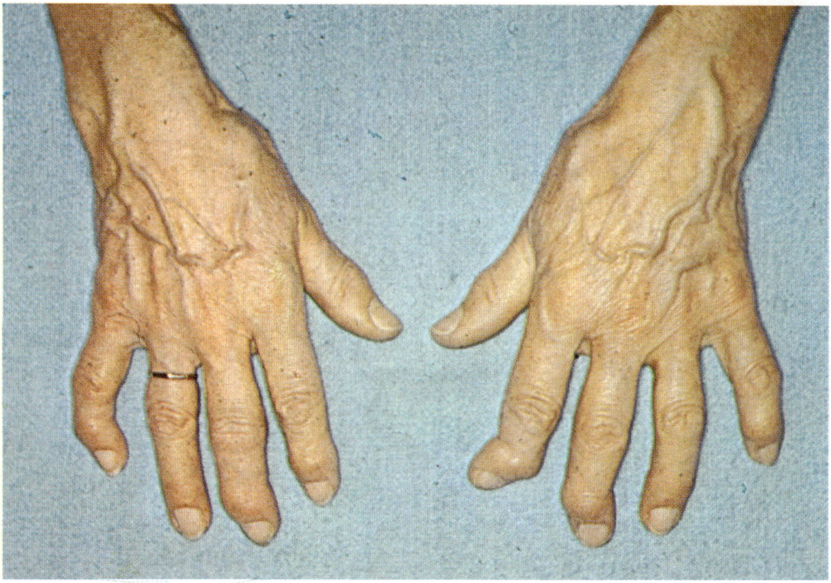

136 Involvement of the proximal interphalangeal joints by osteoarthrosis is less common, the associated swellings being known as Bouchard's nodes, as seen here particularly affecting the fingers of the right hand. Early Heberden's nodes are also present in the thumbs and index fingers.

137 Heberden's and Bouchard's nodes: X-ray showing both types. The cardinal radiological signs are cartilage thinning, osteophyte formation on the lateral aspects of the joints, and subchondral bone sclerosis.

138 Osteoarthrosis of the first carpometacarpal joint is another common site affecting the hand. The X-ray shows large osteophytes around the joint.

136

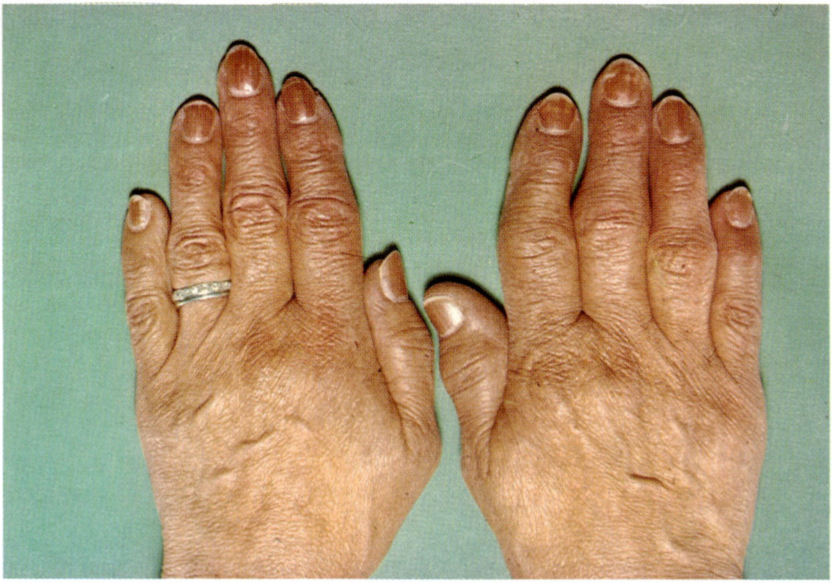

137

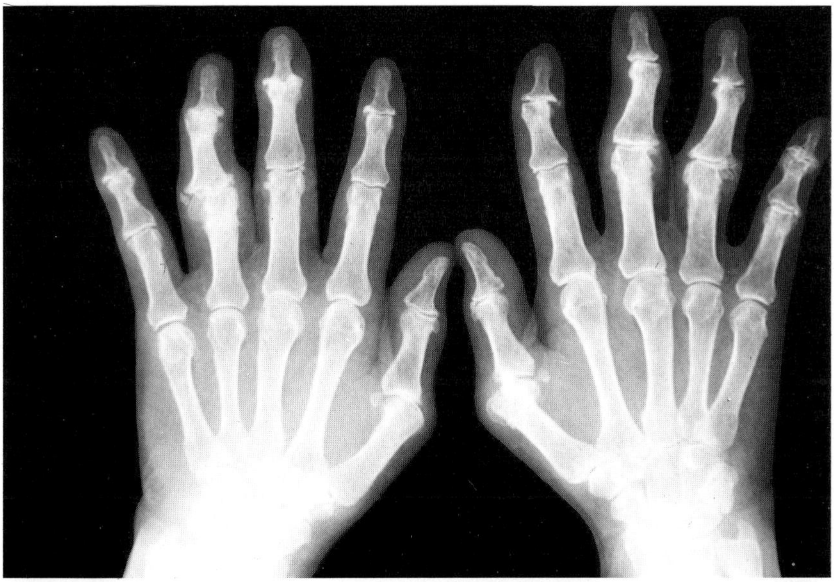

138

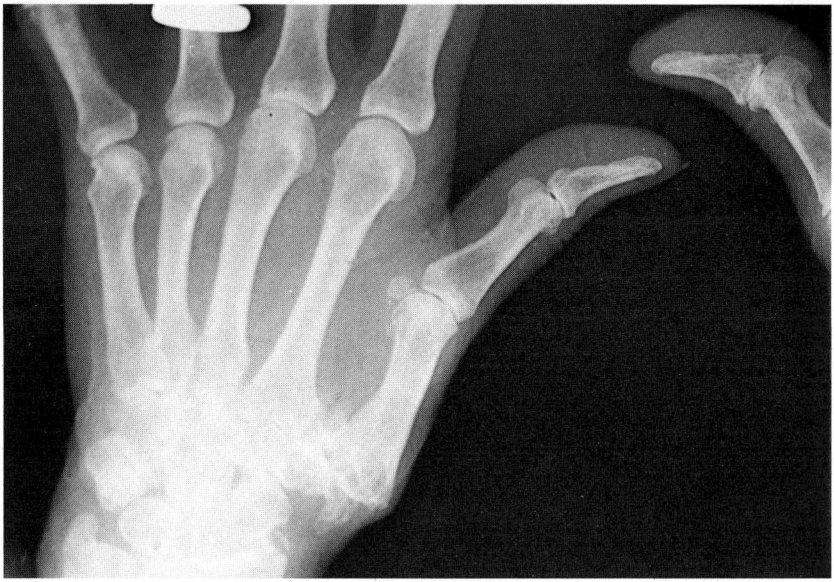

139 Hallux rigidus. The hallux is the most commonly affected joint, resulting in valgus deformity.

140 Early osteoarthrosis of the knee joint. There is cartilage loss in the medial compartment of the joint with early osteophytes on the medial margins of the femoral condyle and tibial plateau. Sharpening of the tibial spines may also be an early radiological feature.

141 More advanced osteoarthrosis of the knee with similar changes affecting both compartments of the joint.

142 Osteoarthrosis affecting the patello-femoral joint shown by lateral X-ray of the knee. Osteophytes are present on the upper pole of the patella, and on the femoral condyle.

143 Severe osteoarthrosis affecting all components of the joint: lateral X-ray. In such cases loose bodies are also common within the joint, and may sometimes cause mechanical locking of the joint.

139

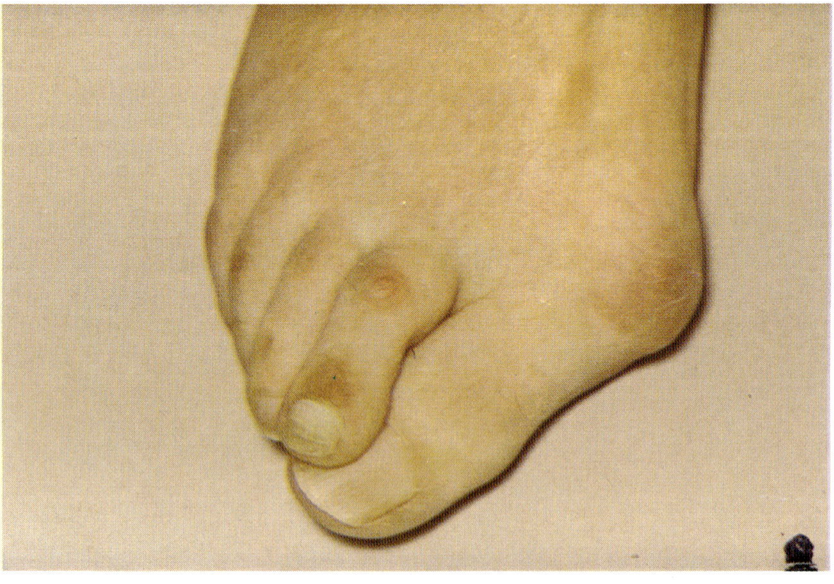

140

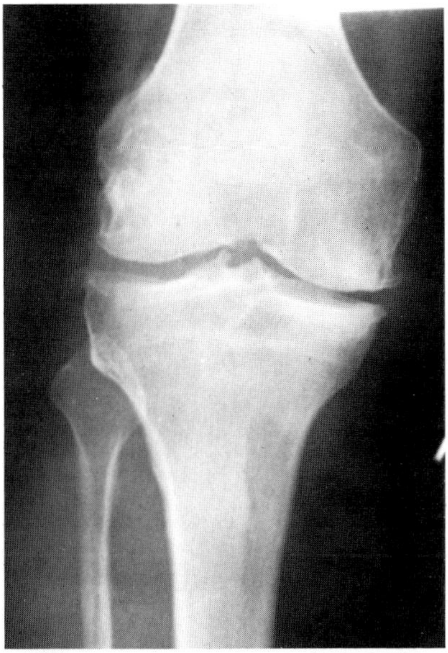

141

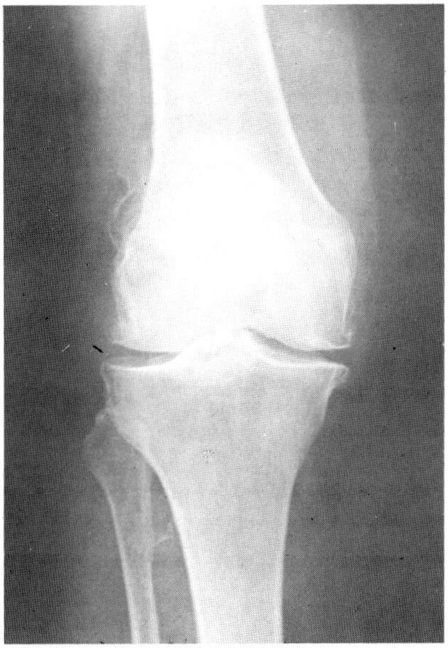

142

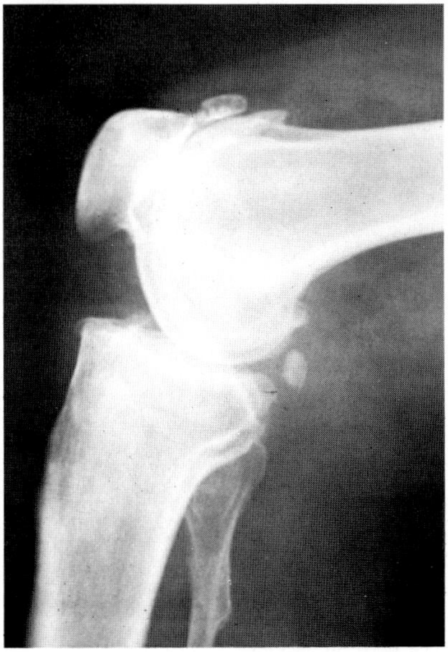

143

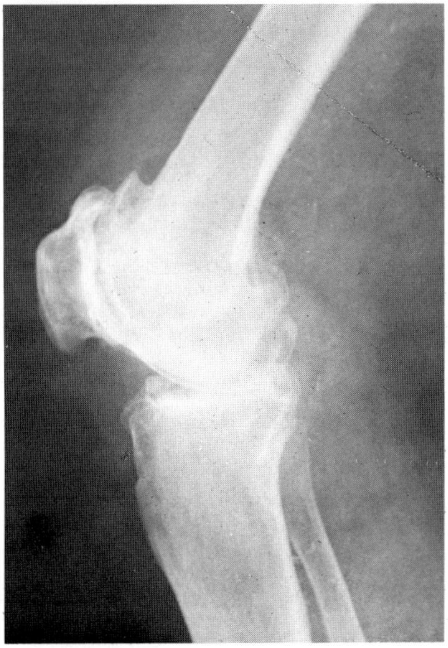

144 Ankle joints are not commonly affected, but when involved give rise to considerable disability.

145 Advanced bilateral osteoarthrosis of the hips. In the right hip there is cartilage thinning and osteophytes around the femoral head. The left hip shows similar changes, but there is partial collapse of the femoral head. This may occur due to cyst formation in the femoral head, weakening the weight bearing surface.

146 Osteoarthrosis of the shoulder. Degenerative changes in shoulders, elbows, wrists and ankles are relatively uncommon and are usually secondary to trauma or other causes.

144

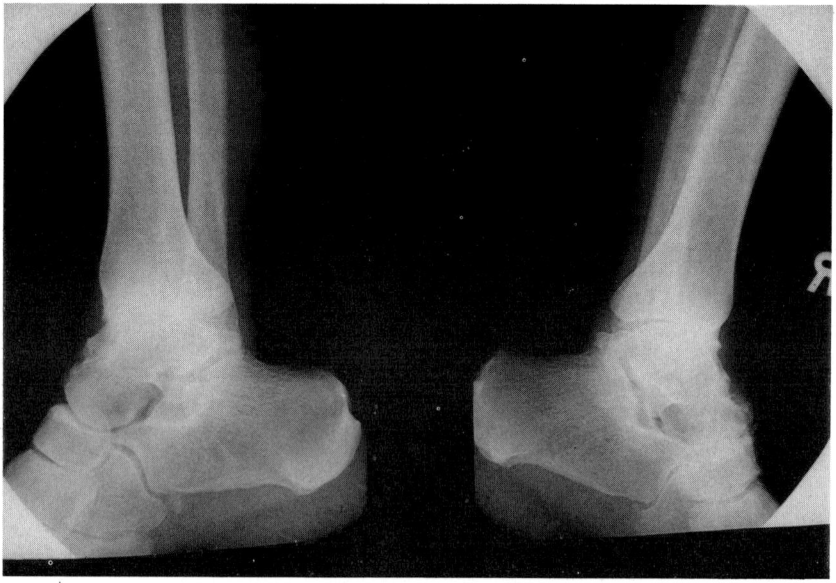

145

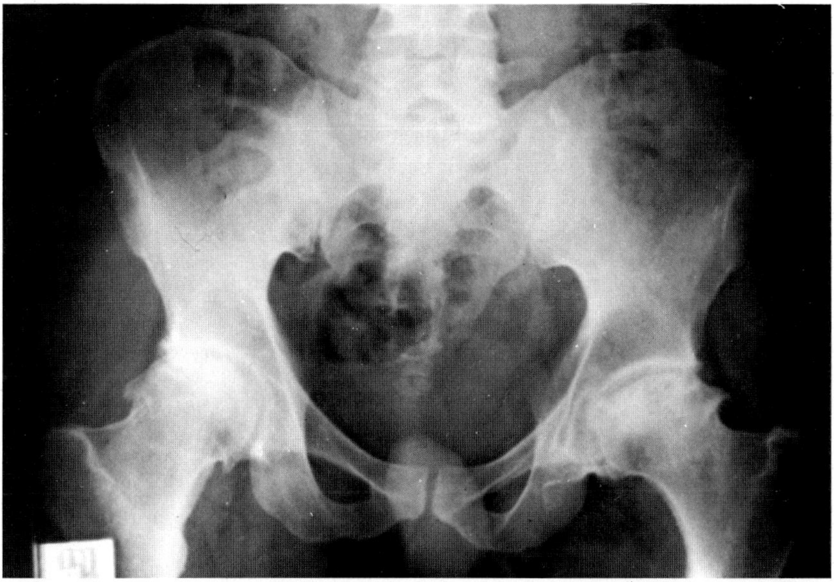

146

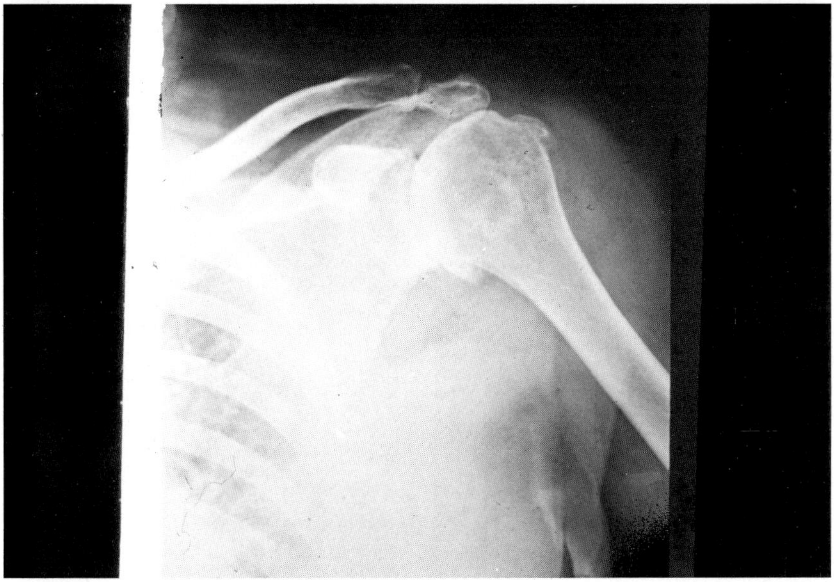

Spondylosis

147 Early degenerative arthritis of the cervical spine (cervical spondylosis). Note narrowing of C5–6 disc with osteophytes on anterior border of adjacent vertebrae.

148 Advanced cervical spondylosis. Generalized disc degeneration has occurred. In the presence of cervical stenosis, cord compression may occur, giving rise to long tract signs involving the lateral and posterior columns.

149 Severe degenerative change in the cervical spine may give rise to subluxation.

150 Myelogram of same patient (**149**).

151 Dorsal spondylosis. Large osteophytes in the lower dorsal segment have fused.

152 Lumbar spondylosis. There is generalized disc degeneration and osteophytes.

147

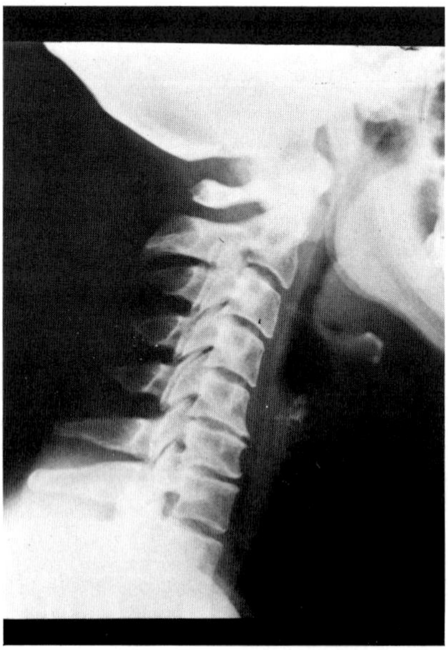

148

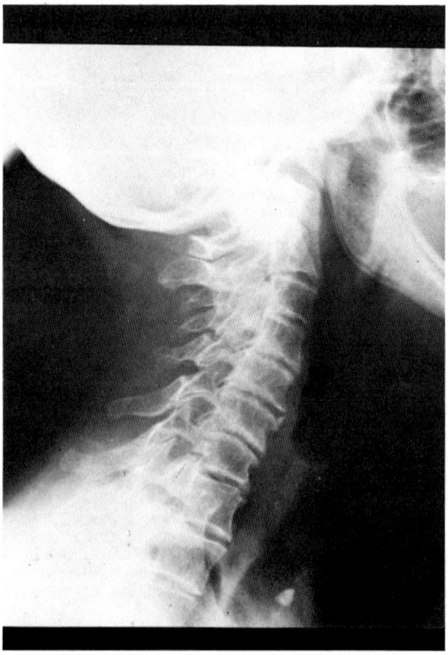

149

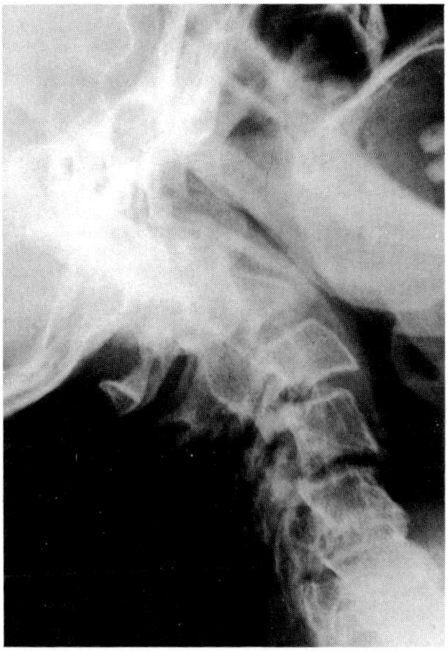

150

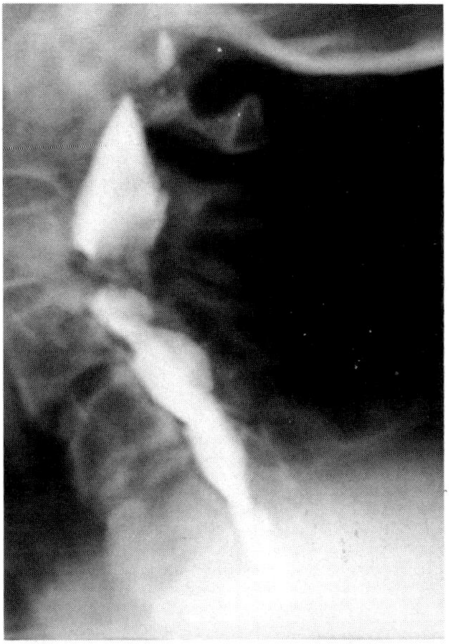

151

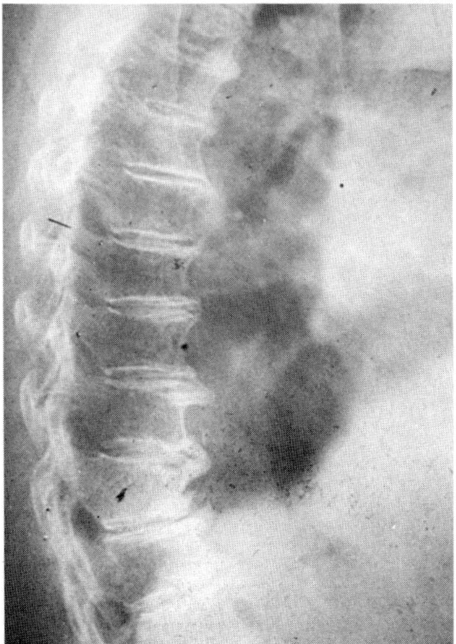

152

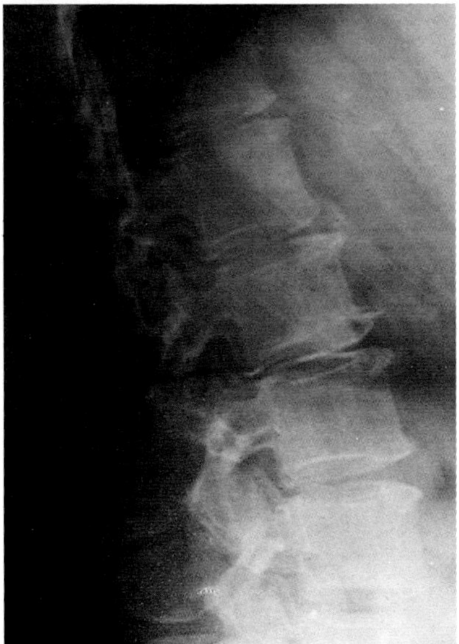

5 Crystal synovitis

There are two common forms of crystal induced synovitis – gout, and chondrocalcinosis (pseudo-gout or calcium gout).

Gout may be primary with a positive family history in 60% of cases, or secondary to other diseases e.g. the myeloproliferative disorders or renal failure. Certain drugs may also cause hyperuricaemia such as a low dosage of salicylates or the thiazide diuretics.

The underlying cause of hyperuricaemia in primary gout is uncertain. Some individuals may be over-producers of urate, some may be under-excretors, but a combination of these two factors may not be uncommon. Familial hyperuricaemia may not necessarily lead to attacks of gout, but the liability to gouty arthritis is directly related to the severity of the hyperuricaemia. Males are affected many times more frequently than females, and acute attacks of gout are uncommon before the fourth decade.

Acute gout most commonly affects the metatarsophalangeal joint of the great toe although any joint may be so affected. Pain is usually much more severe than in other types of inflammatory arthritis, but even if left untreated the attack will almost always subside within 2–3 weeks. Repeated attacks of gout over many years may lead to tophaceous deposits around affected joints or in cartilage (e.g. the ear). If untreated these deposits will eventually cause destructive changes in articular cartilage and may erode underlying bone.

Acute attacks of gout result from the deposition of uric acid crystals within a joint resulting in an acute inflammatory reaction, although why this should occur from time to time remains obscure. Provocative factors in inducing acute gouty arthritis appear to include trauma to a joint, dietary or alcoholic excesses, surgical operations, and the intake of certain drugs.

The clinical picture is usually that of an extremely acute monarthritis, and this, together with the finding of a raised serum uric acid, is usually sufficient to make a firm diagnosis. In cases of doubt, a definite diagnosis may be made by aspirating an affected joint (or needling a tophus), and identifying crystals of uric acid under polarised light microscopy.

Renal disease is the most frequent complication of gout, and may vary from a mild proteinuria to the deposition of urates within the kidney with vascular changes or pyelonephritis. In addition, there is some evidence of an increased liability to hypertension and arterial disease in those patients with significantly raised levels of serum uric acid.

Chondrocalcinosis (pseudo-gout, or calcium gout) is another form of crystal synovitis, less common than uric acid gout, and due to the local deposition of crystals of calcium pyrophosphate dihydrate. As in true gout, the typical crystals may be identified in joint fluid or within leucocytes. The metabolic disturbance underlying the disease is unknown, but it may be associated with uric acid gout, hypertension, diabetes mellitus, or hyperparathyroidism. In cases not associated with other conditions, biochemical studies are remarkable for their normality.

Unlike uric acid gout, males are not predominantly affected: the clinical picture of an acute inflammatory mon-arthritis closely resembles true gout but larger joints – usually the knees or wrists – are most commonly affected. Occasionally the condition presents as an acute polyarthritis resembling rheumatoid arthritis, or may give rise to premature and widespread degenerative arthritis. In a small proportion of cases there appears to be a hereditary factor.

The diagnosis should be suspected in any middle aged woman who develops a sudden and acute inflammatory arthritis of one or other knee joint. It can be confirmed by aspiration of the affected joint and finding the typical weakly positive birefringent crystals in the joint fluid, or by the radiological exhibition of calcification within joint menisci or articular cartilage.

Apart from chondrocalcinosis, calcification of articular cartilage may be seen in other conditions – notably following renal dialysis.

Gout

153 Crystals of uric acid in a joint fluid aspirate seen under polarised light microscopy.

154 Acute gout affecting the left 1st metatarsophalangeal joint. Intense inflammatory changes with oedema have spread to involve the whole foot. Exquisite tenderness is a marked clinical feature.

155 Resolving attack of gout in the left hallux. Inflammatory changes and oedema are subsiding. Previous attacks have lead to discolouration and distortion of the right hallux.

156 Close-up view of the same patient (**155**).

153

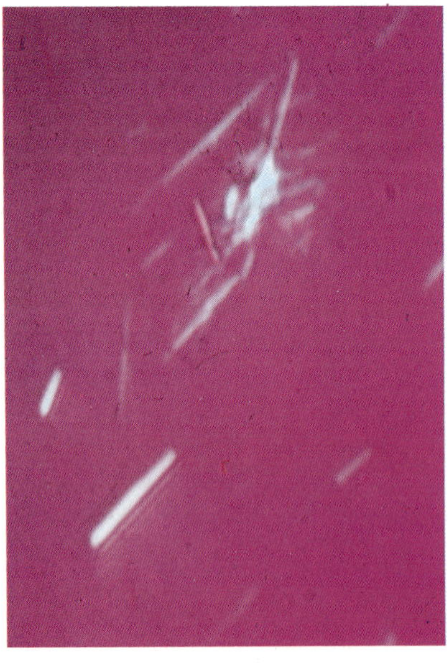

154

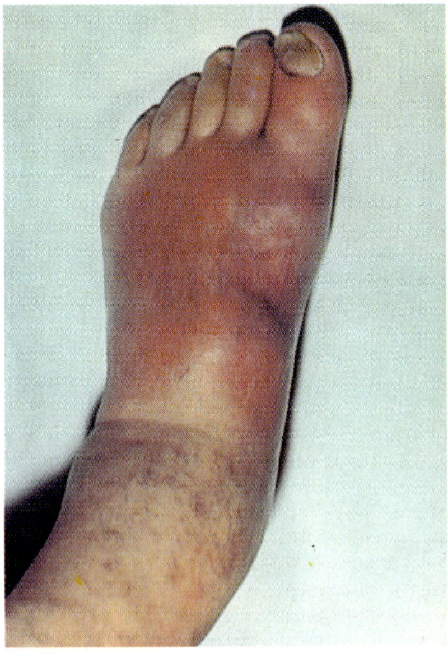

155

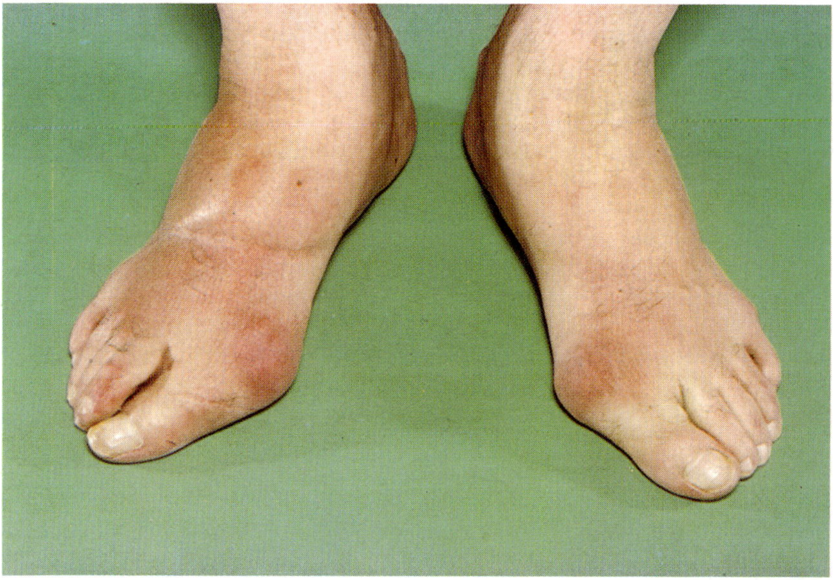

156

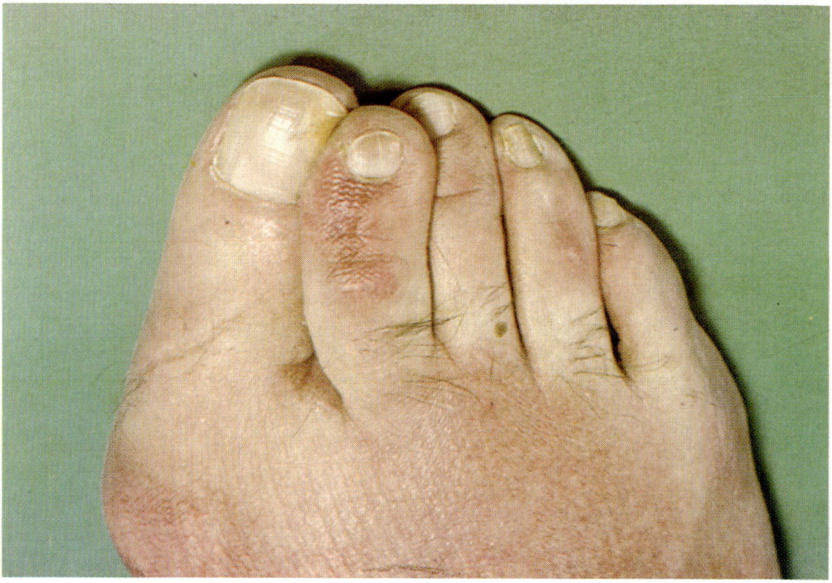

157 Repeated attacks may eventually lead to a continuing low grade inflammation with destructive changes as seen in the left hallux.

158 Chronic gouty arthritis affecting both hallux joints. On the left, residual deposits of urate give rise to a large soft tissue swelling around the joint and ulceration of urate into bone is shown as the large 'punched out' area in the head of the 1st metatarsal.

159 Chronic gouty arthritis affecting the finger joints. Large deposits of urate remain around the terminal joint of the thumb, and the proximal interphalangeal joints of the middle and little fingers.

160 Chronic gout in halluces.

157

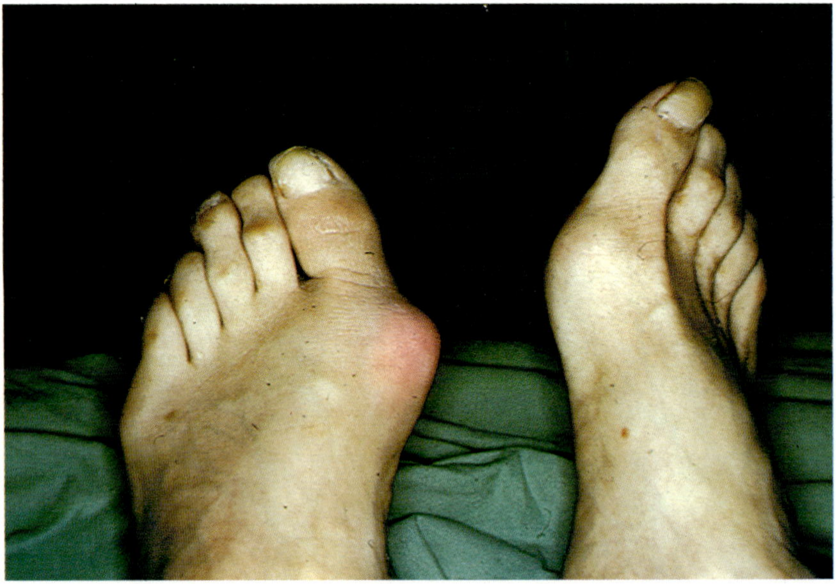

158

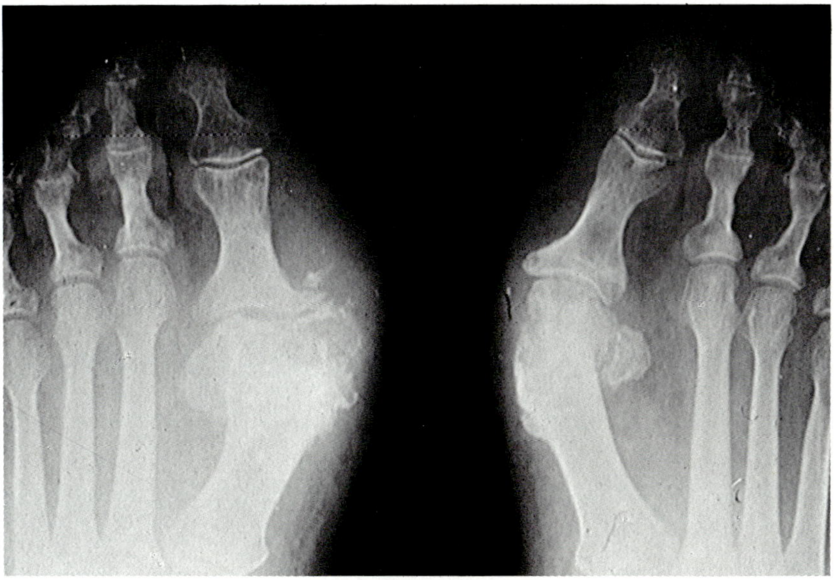

159

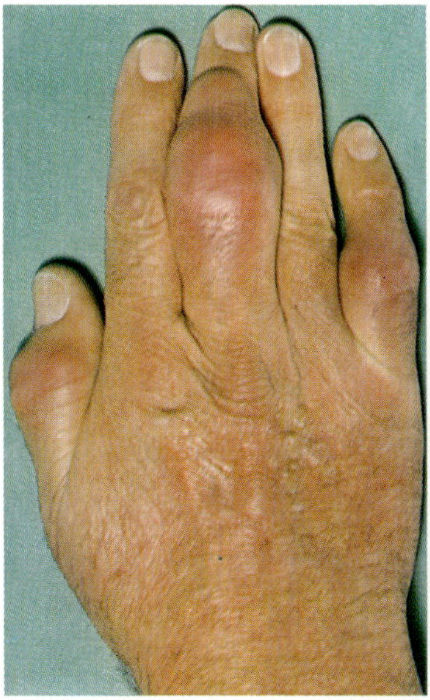

160

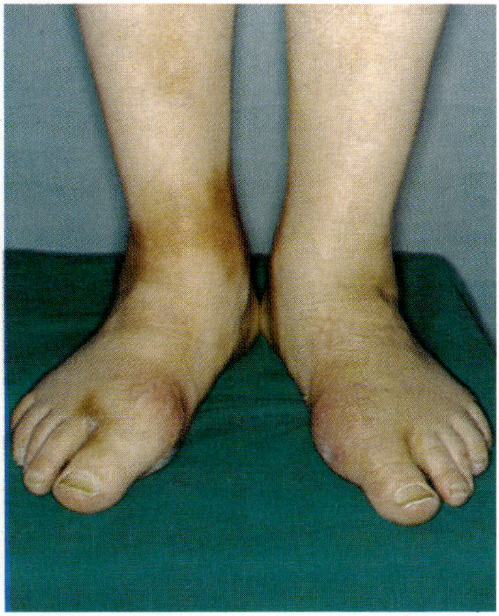

161 Chronic gouty arthritis: X-ray of the hands of a patient with this disease. Multiple punched out areas are seen due to urate deposition.

162 Bursae may also be the seat of deposition of urate crystals causing acute inflammation. This picture shows acute right olecranon bursitis.

163 Acute pre-patellar bursitis due to gout.

161

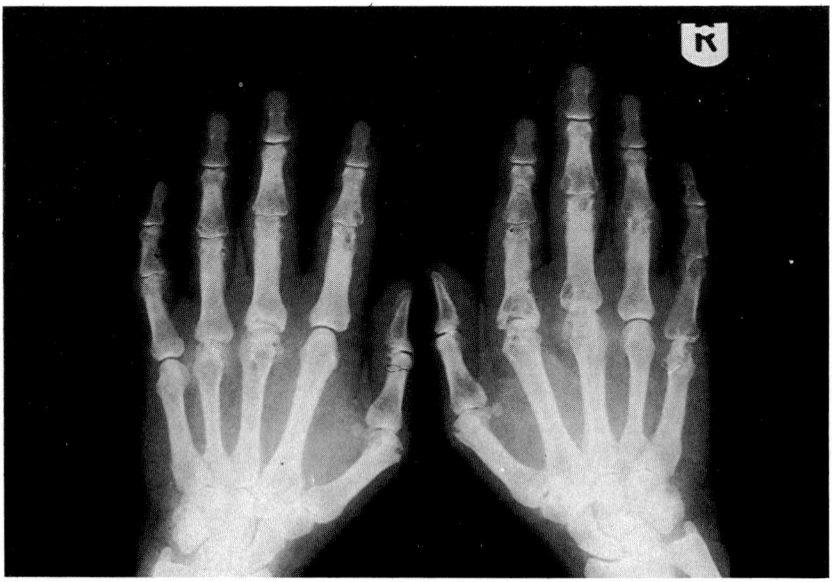

162

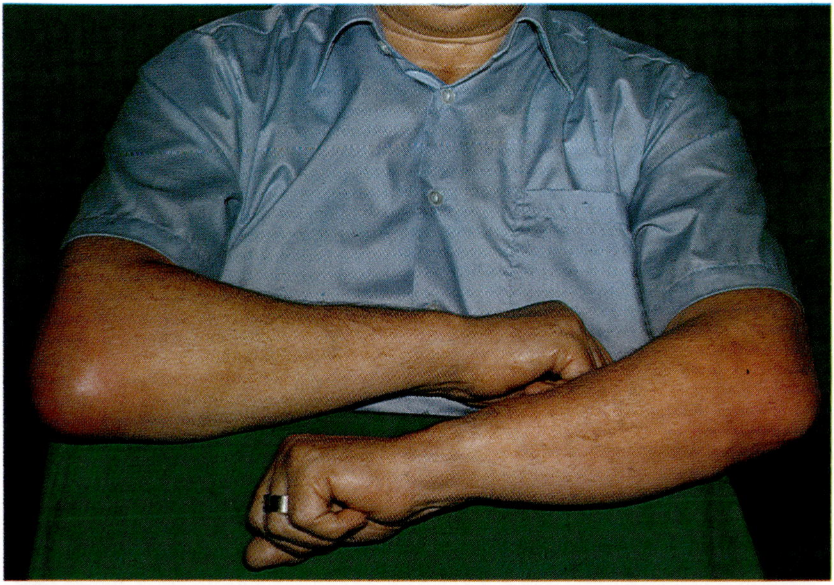

163

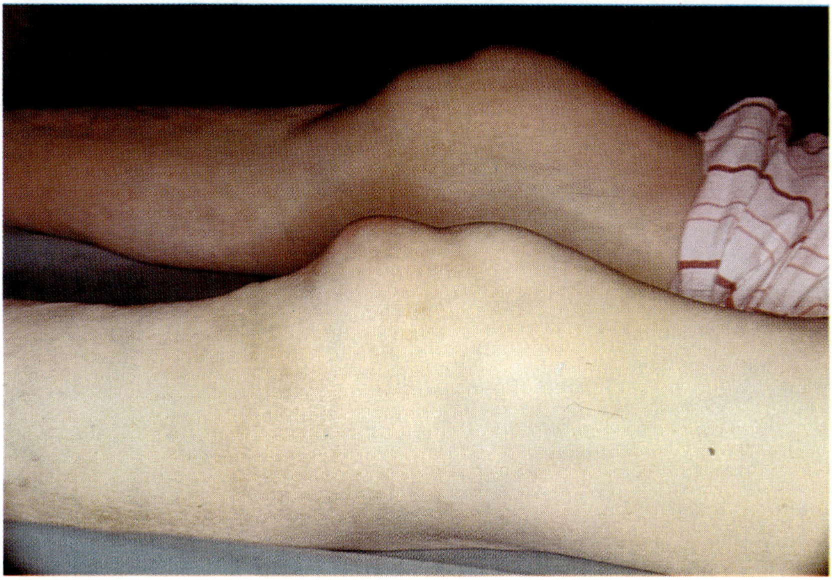

164 Chronic gouty olecranon bursitis.

165 Tophaceous urate deposits may occur in cartilage, particularly the ear. An early tophus can just be seen at '10 o'clock' in this ear.

166 Early tophus: a close-up view.

167 Large tophaceous deposits in chronic longstanding gout.

168 Tophus in a finger joint.

164

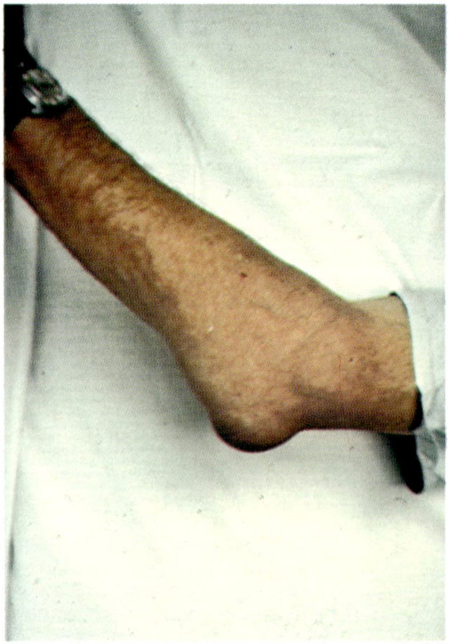

165

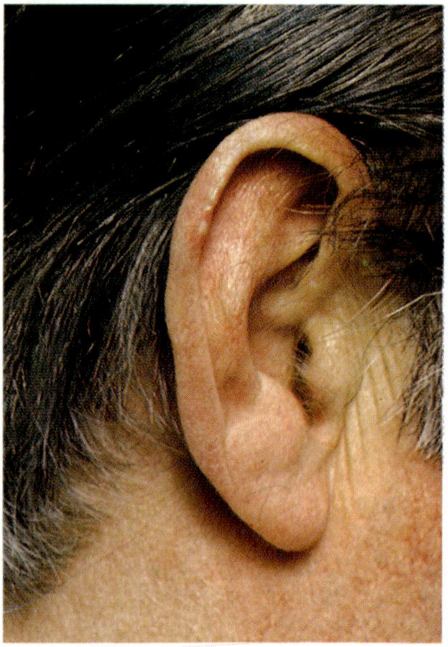

166

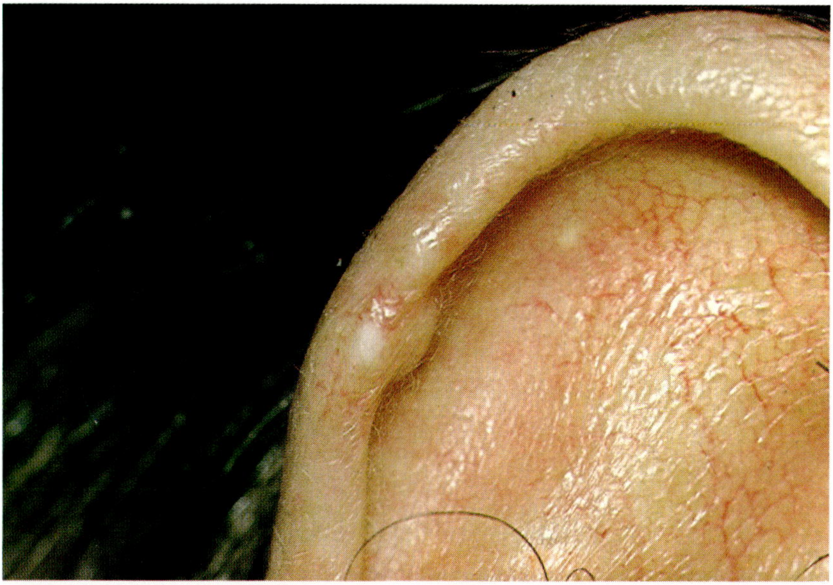

167

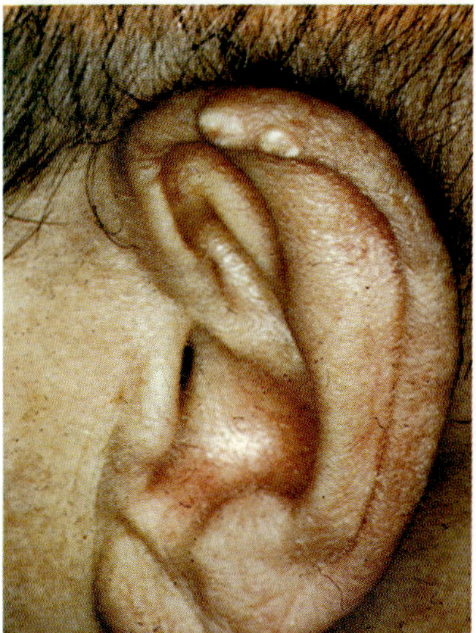

168

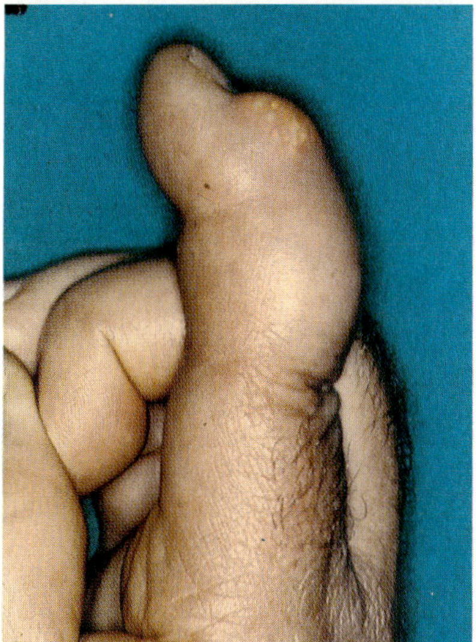

169 Knee joint in chondrocalcinosis: characteristic X-ray appearance. Calcification is seen in both menisci in the antero-posterior view, while in the lateral view a thin rim of calcification is seen in the articular cartilage on the posterior aspect of the femoral condyle.

170 The calcification in the articular cartilage of the femoral condyle is shown in enlarged view of same patient (**169**).

171 The wrist in chondrocalcinosis. Calcification is seen in the triangular ligament

169

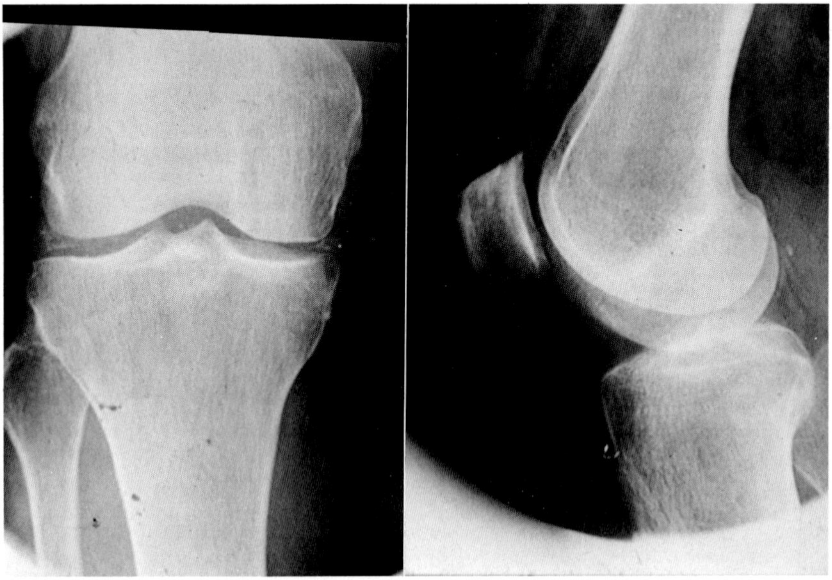

170

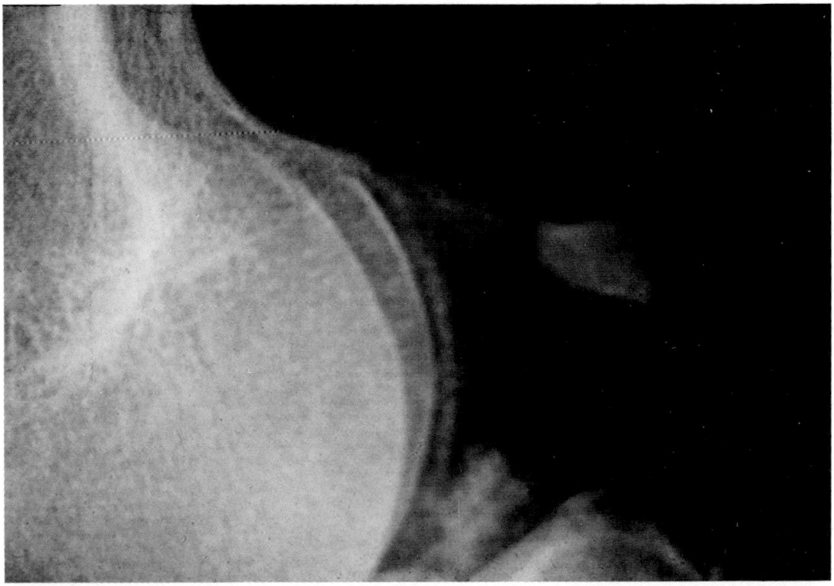

171

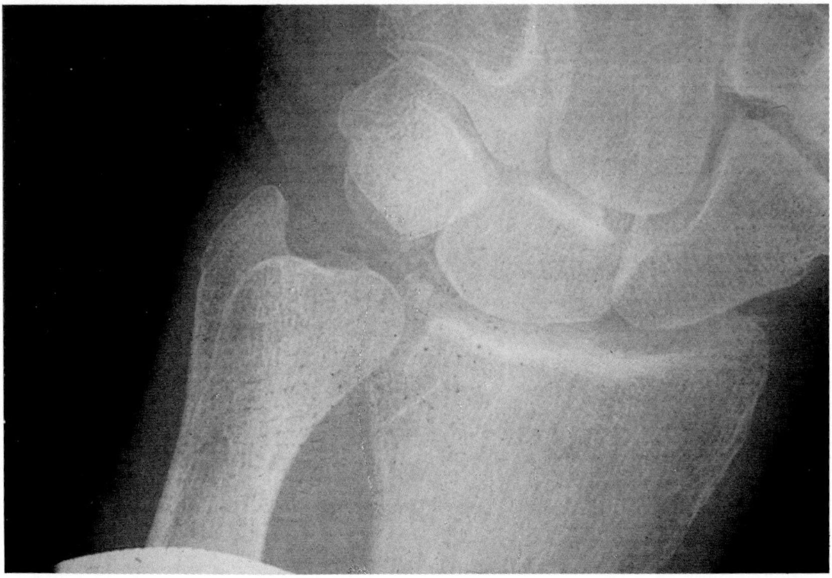

PATTERNS OF ARTHRITIS IN CHONDROCALCINOSIS

Type A *Pseudogout:* Monoarticular inflammatory episodes
Type B *Pseudo RA:* Symmetrical inflammatory polyarthritis
Type C *Acute or chronic arthritis* of larger weight-bearing joints (i.e. lumbar spine; hip; and knee)
Type D *Chronic progressive arthritis:* same joints as type C
Type E *Asymptomatic*

172

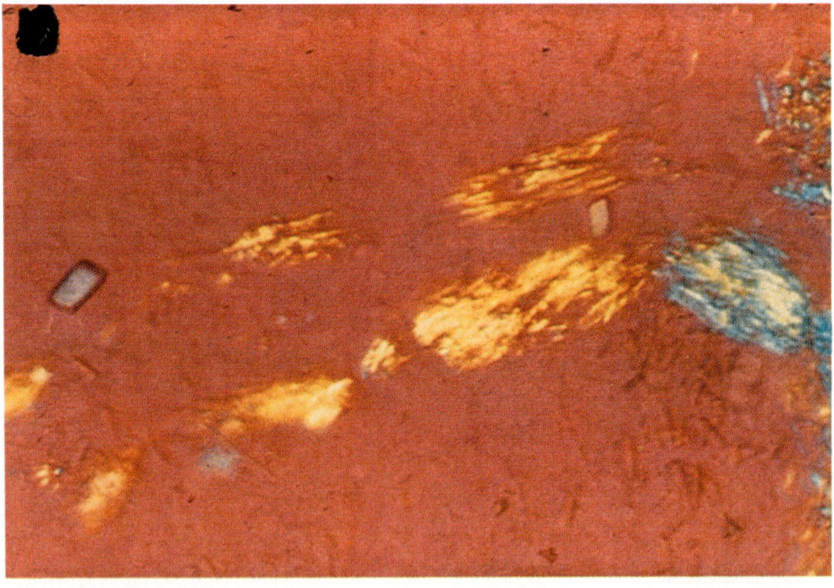

172 Rhomboidal crystals of calcium pyrophosphate dihydrate ingested by leucocytes, seen in the aspirate from an affected joint under polarised light microscopy.

6 Connective tissue disorders

In the following chapter are illustrated four of the more important connective tissue disorders – systemic lupus erythematosus, systemic sclerosis, polyarteritis nodosa, and polymyositis or dermatomyositis.

More recently an entity known as 'mixed connective tissue disease' has been recognised. As the name would suggest, this disorder has features which overlap the other diseases in the group.

Connective tissue is composed essentially of collagen, elastic fibres and fibroblasts in an amorphous ground substance. A common thread is seen to run through the histological changes in these diseases, particularly the widespread vascular pathology and the fibrinoid change in the ground substance. Consequently they have many clinical features in common, and it is not always possible to decide with certainty into which diagnostic category a patient may fall.

With the exception of progressive systemic sclerosis the advent of steroid therapy has vastly improved the prognosis of these diseases which previously resulted so often in a fatal outcome.

Each is a multi-system disease with a widely variable clinical picture, but the major features of each (there are many others), may be summarised as follows:

Systemic lupus erythematosus: fever, arthralgia or arthritis, skin rashes, proteinuria, polyserositis, hepatosplenomegaly, and neuro-psychiatric disturbances.

Progressive systemic sclerosis: thickening of the skin and telangiectasia, Raynaud's phenomenon, dysphagia, subcutaneous calcinosis, and renal failure.

Polyarteritis nodosa: fever, muscle and joint pains, bronchial asthma, abdominal pain, hypertension, renal disease, and mononeuritis multiplex.

Polymyositis or dermatomyositis: profound proximal muscle weakness, muscle pain and tenderness, arthralgia or arthritis, dusky erythema of the face, upper arms and thorax, and violaceous discoloration around nail beds.

Mixed connective tissue disease: this 'overlap syndrome' may present with features predominantly like systemic lupus erythematosus, or progressive systemic sclerosis, but any features of either may be present, together with myositis. However, renal involvement is usually either mild or absent thus making the prognosis much better than in the other diseases in the group.

The illustrations which follow show some of the more important clinical and histological features of these diseases.

Systemic lupus erythematosus

SLE is a multi-system disease which may present in a variety of ways. The most constant features are fever, arthralgia or arthritis, skin rashes, and polyserositis. There is no constant pattern of the disease and diagnosis may be difficult.

The pattern of joint symptoms and signs is variable, sometimes presenting as a flitting mono- or polyarthritis, and sometimes being clinically indistinguishable from rheumatoid arthritis. Often the degree of pain complained of by the patient is much more than would be expected from the physician's examination – a feature which should lead one to suspect the disease.

The butterfly rash on the face is the most typical skin manifestation, but non-specific or petechial rashes may also occur on other parts of the body. Alopecia, localised or generalised, may occur.

Episodes of chest pain, in the absence of either clinical or radiological signs, may occur. Pleural and peri-cardial effusions signify a polyserositis, and myocarditis or aortic insufficiency may lead to cardiac failure.

Psychoses or actual fits may occur, but peripheral neuropathies are less common than in rheumatoid arthritis.

The most serious feature of the disease is renal involvement, usually heralded by the advent of proteinuria, and if progressive, it may determine a fatal outcome. It is found in about 75% of cases coming to autopsy.

Certain drugs are known to induce an SLE-like syndrome, among the most important of which are: procainamide; hydrallazine; anticonvulsants; and isoniazid. Many other drugs have been suspected (D-Penicillamine, oral contraceptives etc.) but direct proof is lacking.

173

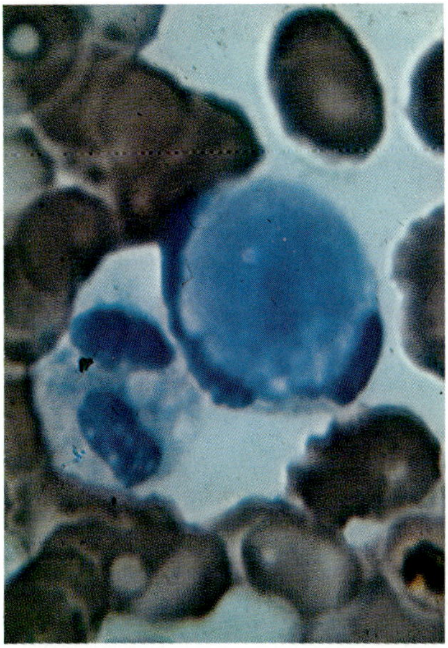

173 The LE cell (seen here) is only found in about 75% of cases, and a more reliable test is for antinuclear antibody which is positive in 95% of patients with active disease.

174 Antinuclear antibody in SLE shown by immunofluorescence.

174

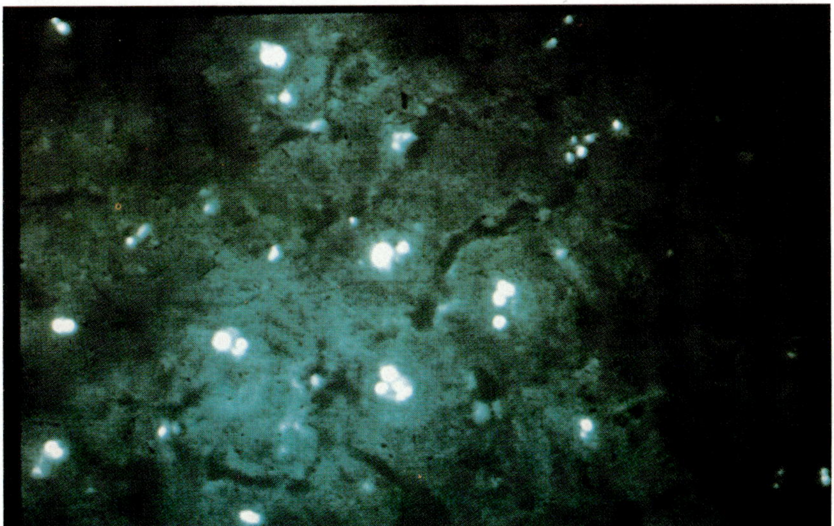

175 'Butterfly rash' is the most common skin manifestation of SLE. This is a sunlight sensitive rash occurring over the bridge of the nose and cheeks. Note the bullous eruption around the lips.

176 'Persistent sunburn effect'. The forearms and other areas exposed to sunlight may be affected, giving this effect.

177 SLE: X-ray of the hands of a patient with this disease. Severe pain in the joints may be present for many years, yet destruction of cartilage and bone, as in rheumatoid arthritis is rarely seen.

MARKERS OF AUTO-IMMUNE DISEASE

1. Increased production of immunoglobulins
2. Demonstrable autoantibodies against tissue components
3. Deposition of altered gamma globulins in tissues
4. Proliferation of lymphoid and plasma cells
5. Multiplicity of immune manifestations
6. Response to corticosteroids and immunosuppressive agents

175

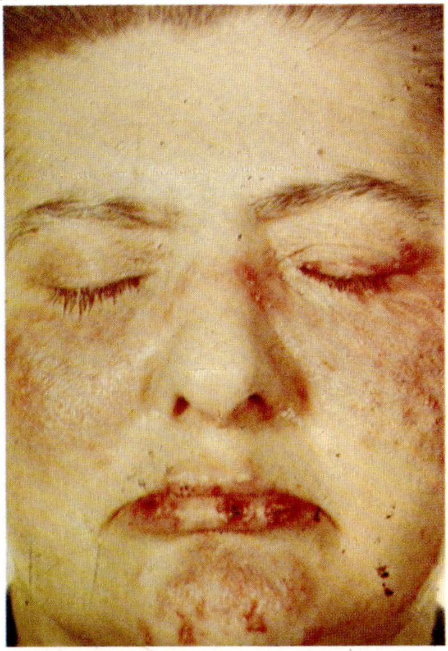

176

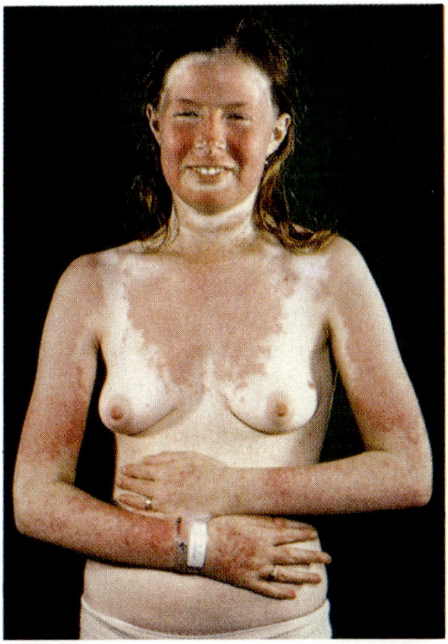

177

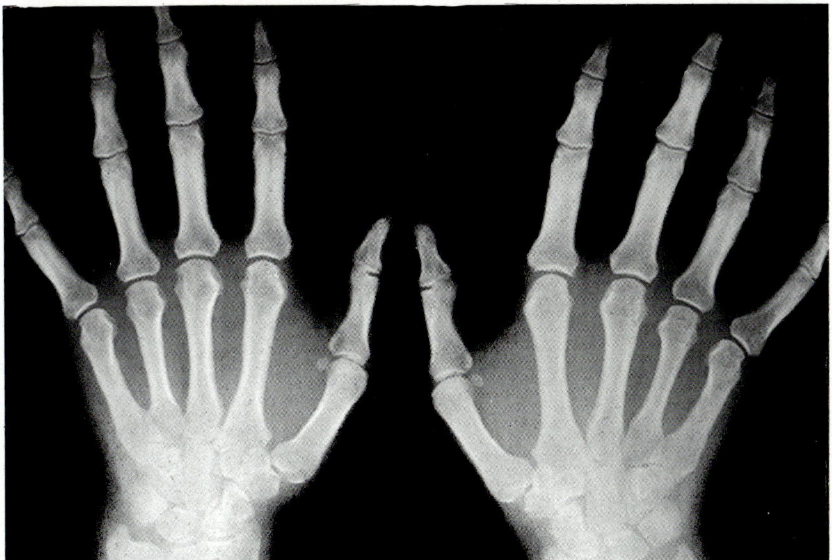

178 SLE retinopathy. Exudates occur in the absence of other causes and are known as 'cytoid bodies'.

179 The 'wire loop' lesion. Focal glomerulitis is followed by an increase in the thickness of the basement membrane and tubular degeneration. The final picture is that of chronic glomerulo-nephritis. Many patients develop a protein-losing kidney of the nephrotic syndrome type, while others may have a pyelonephritis which may be mistaken for SLE nephritis. (× *150*)

180 The spleen in SLE showing the 'onion skin' appearance, due to peri-arterial fibrosis. (× *150*)

178

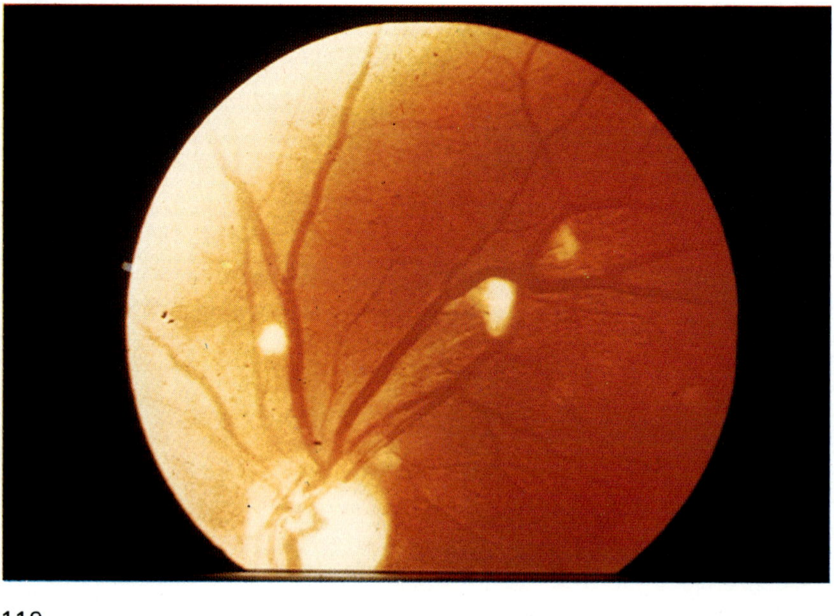

179

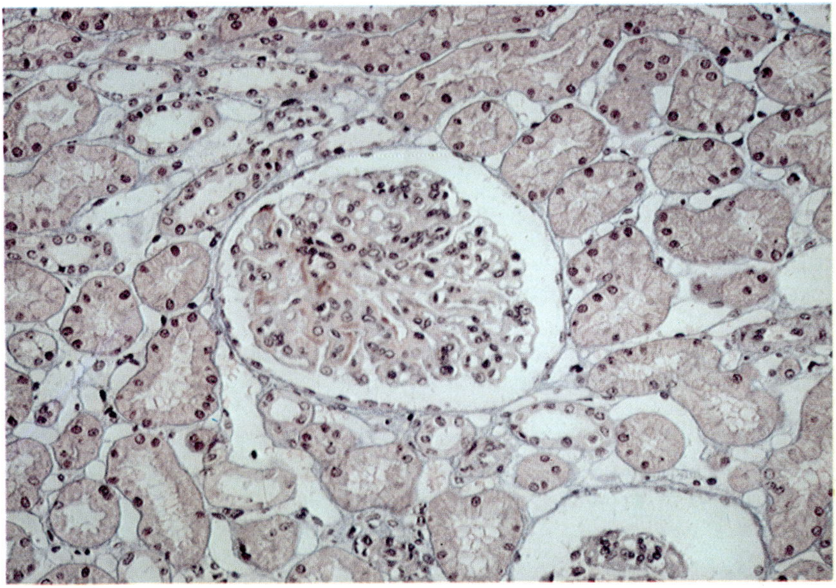

180

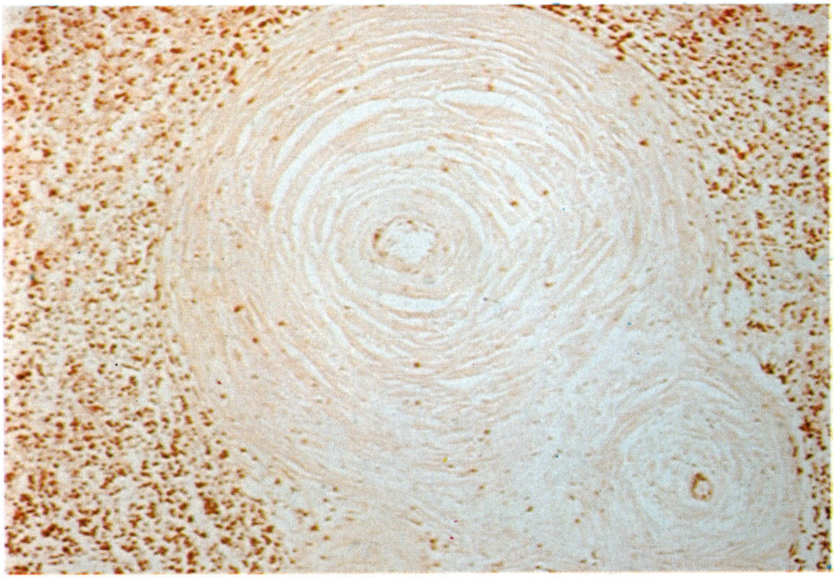

Progressive systemic sclerosis (Scleroderma)

The characteristic features of this disease are thickening of the skin of the extremities, sometimes spreading to the trunk, Raynaud's phenomenon, subcutaneous calcific deposits, and telangiectasis. Like SLE it may progress to a multi-system disease with pulmonary, cardiac, renal, and gastrointestinal manifestations.

Scleroderma may form part of the picture of 'mixed connective tissue disease' (see page 134).

181 Early scleroderma of the fingers. The skin is thickened, waxy in appearance, and bound down to underlying tissue.

182 Scleroderma of hands showing gross limitation of flexion of the fingers due to thickening of the skin.

183 Advanced scleroderma of hands. Necrosis of terminal phalanges has occurred from ischaemia due to Raynaud's phenomenon with fixed flexion deformities of the fingers.

181

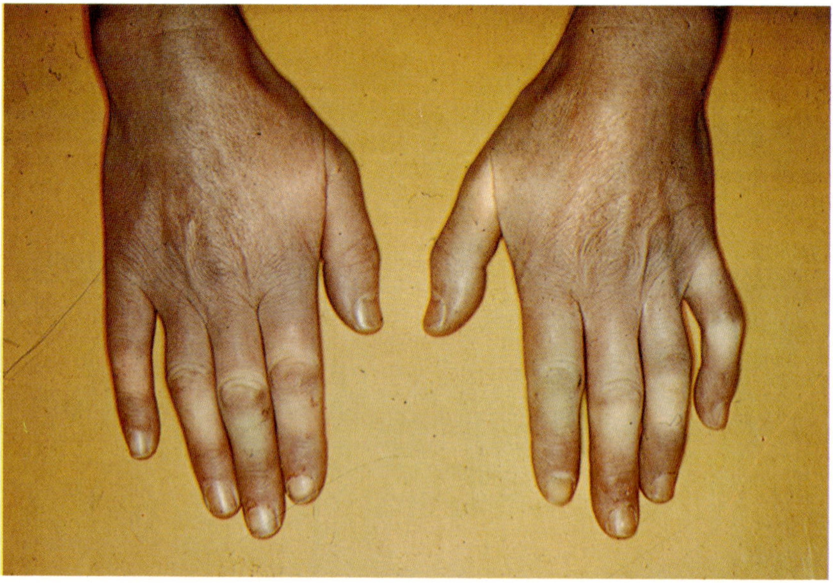

182

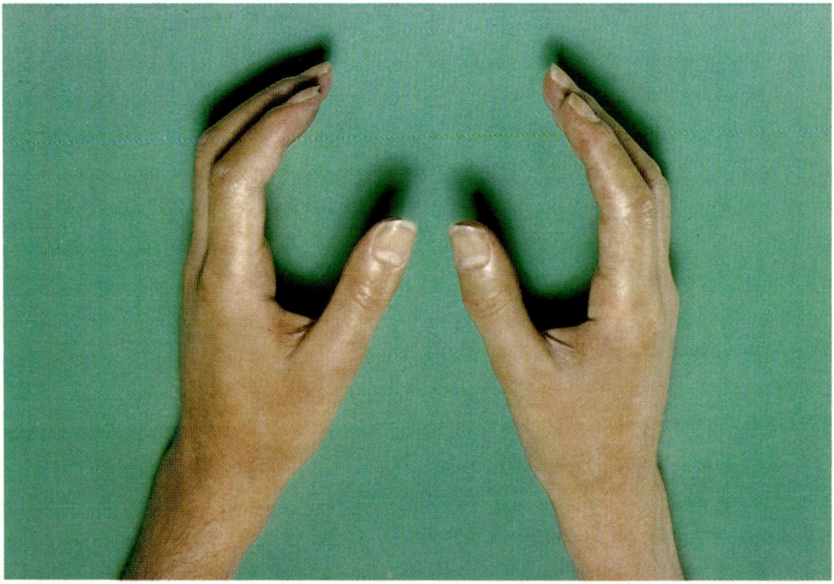

183

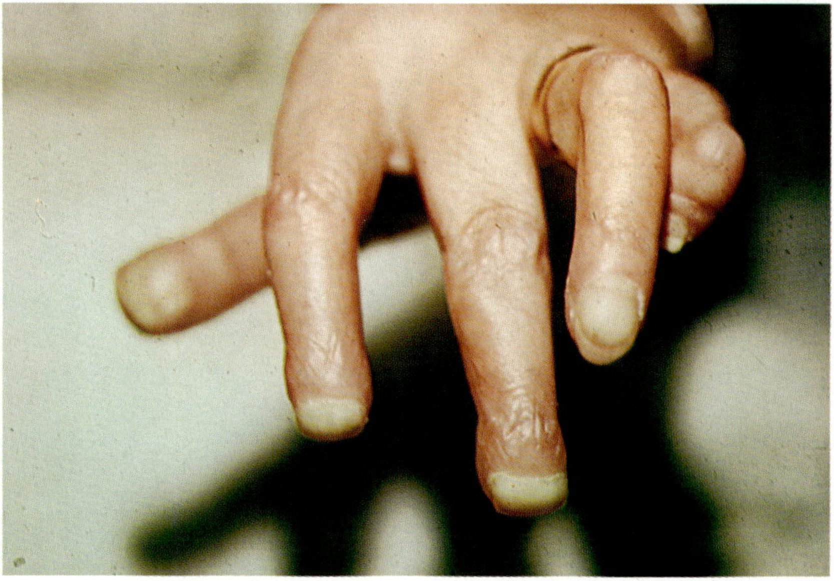

184 Another view of the same hands (**183**). Note the white deposits of calcific material indicating calcinosis.

185 Scleroderma of the upper trunk with thickened, fixed, and shiny skin.

186 Widespread scleroderma affecting hands, trunk and face. There is widespread telangiectasia, and thickened skin around the mouth.

184

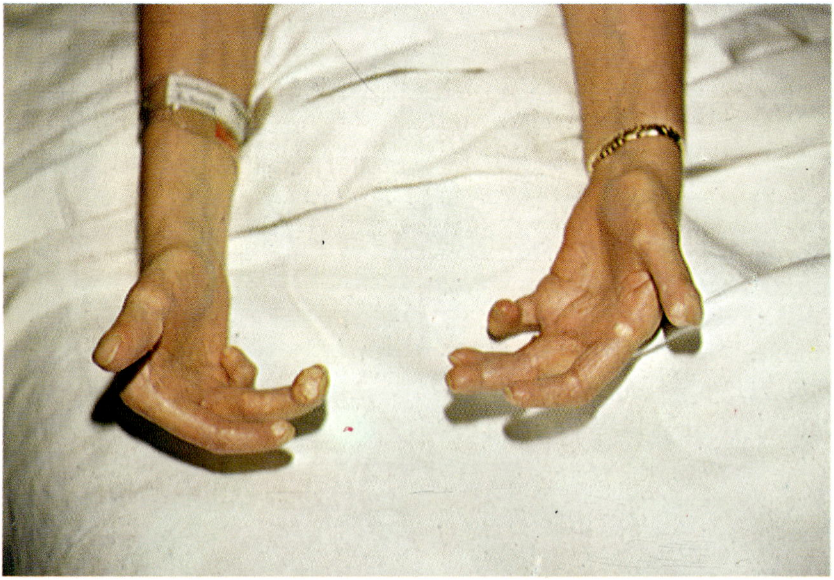

185

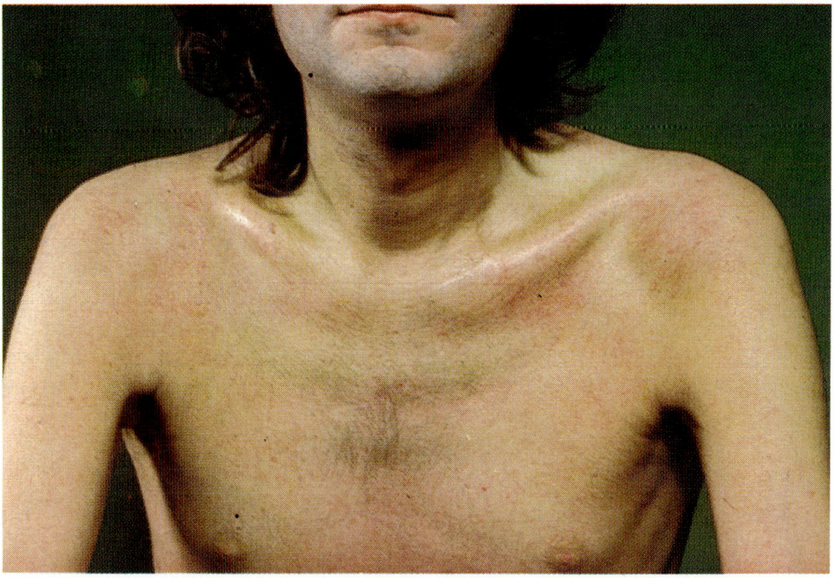

186

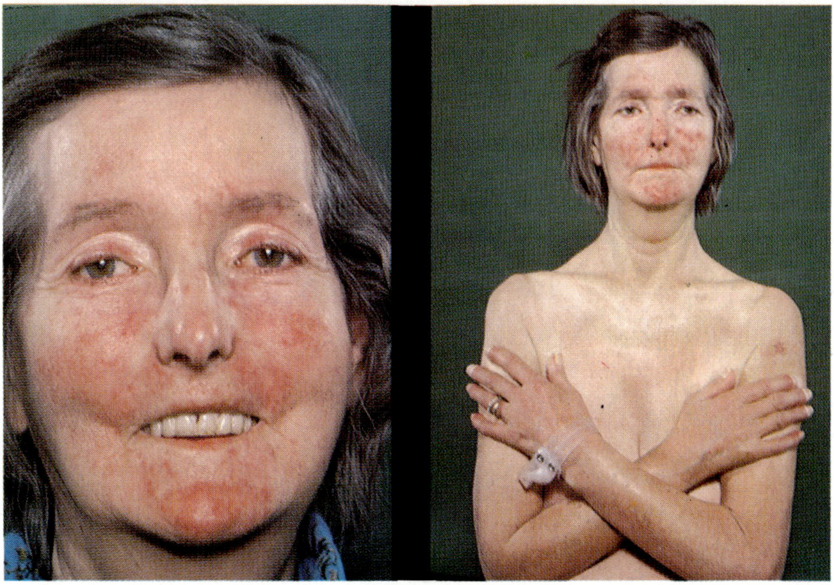

187 The hands in scleroderma: There is (1) necrosis of the phalanx of the right index finger; and (2) early calcific deposits in the pulps of both thumbs.

188 More advanced scleroderma showing necrosis of several terminal phalanges, flexion contractures, and widespread calcific deposits.

189 Dysphagia is common due to involvement of the oesophagus in the fibrotic process. Barium swallow X-ray shows narrowing and lack of peristalsis.

190 Calcinosis in forearm.

187

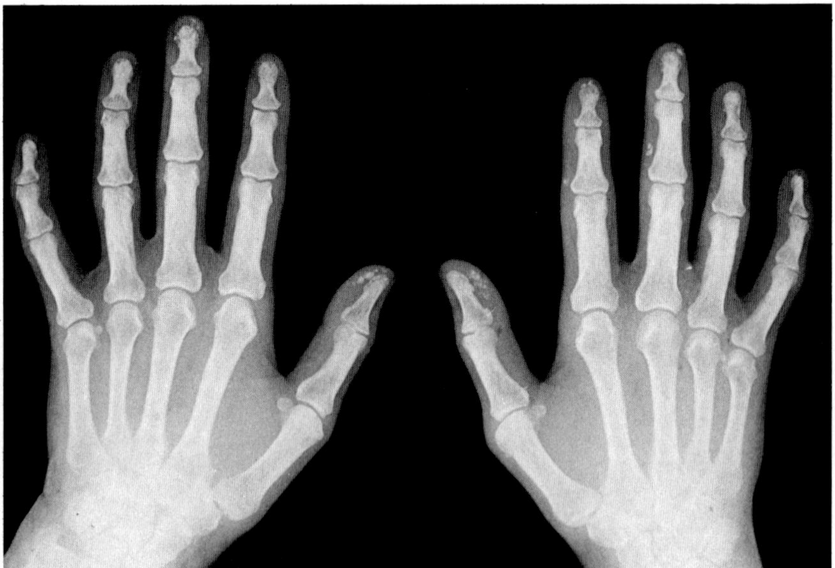

188

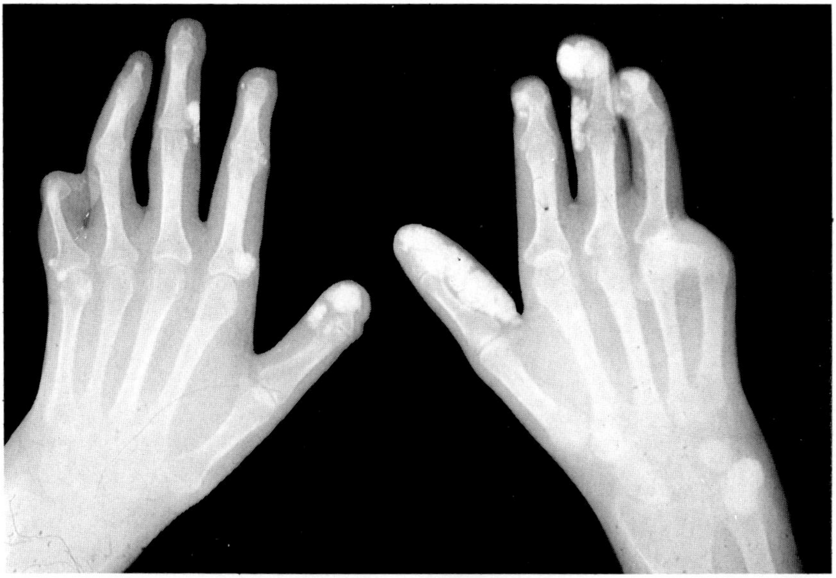

189

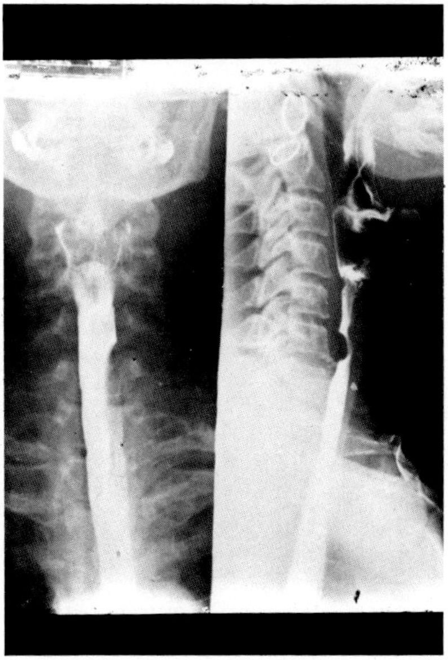

190

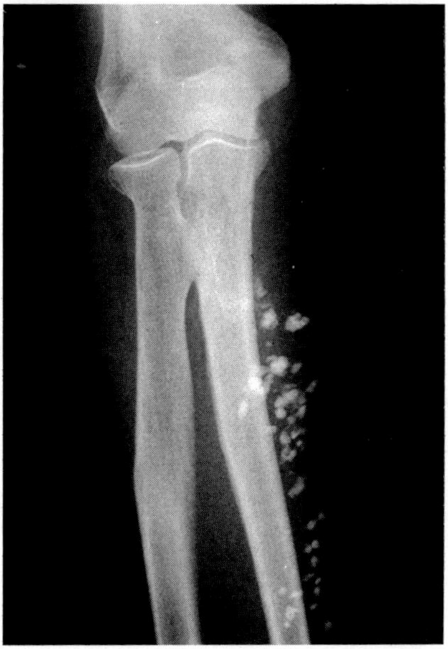

191 Section of kidney in progressive systemic sclerosis. The typical renal lesion is heralded by the onset of a malignant hypertension, rapidly followed by proteinuria and a rising blood urea. The outstanding lesion on microscopical examination is intimal hyperplasia with fibrinoid necrosis of the small arteries leading to occlusion (seen in upper right of illustration). These changes are identical with those found in malignant nephrosclerosis and carry the same serious prognosis. (× *150*)

192 Section of skin in scleroderma. Note loss of rete pegs and dense thickening of dermal collagen, with loss of adnexal structures. Note also that fibrosis extends below the level of the sweat gland seen lower left centre. (× *20*)

193 Fibrosis shown in section of heart muscle.

194 Fibrosis affecting the left ventricle. The heart may be affected, often presenting as a conduction defect.

191

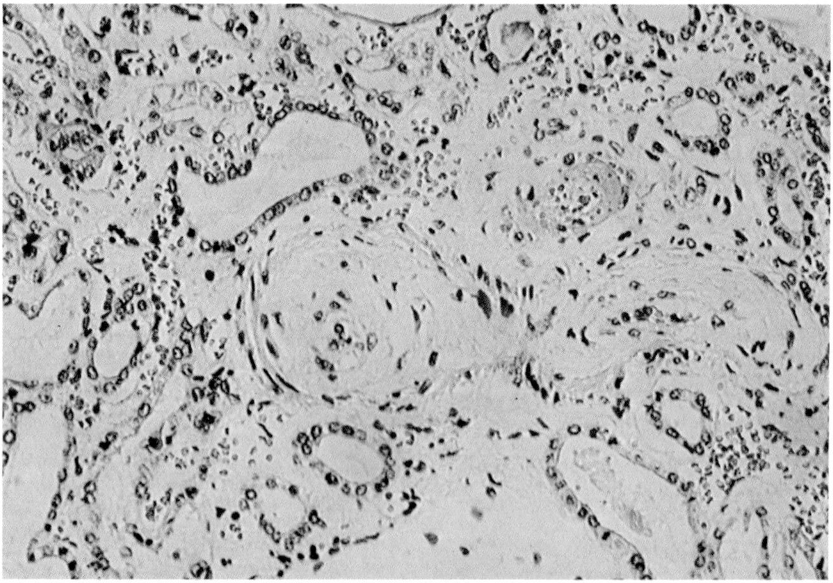

192

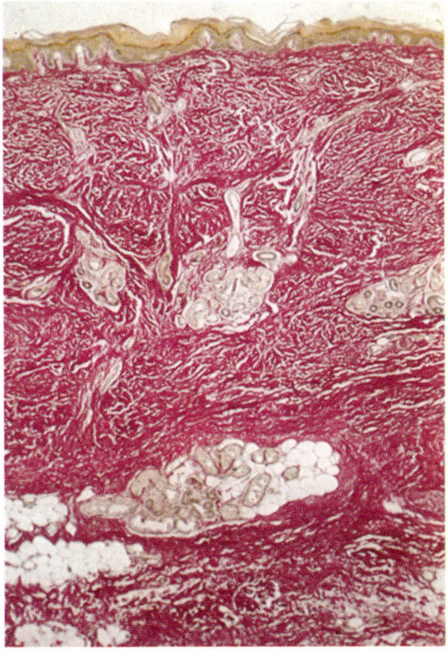

193

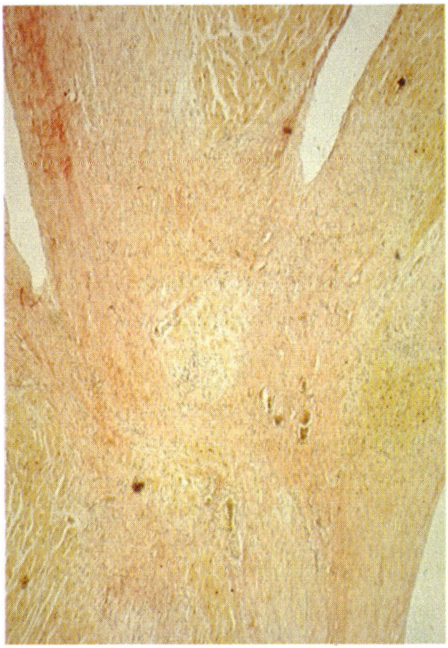

194

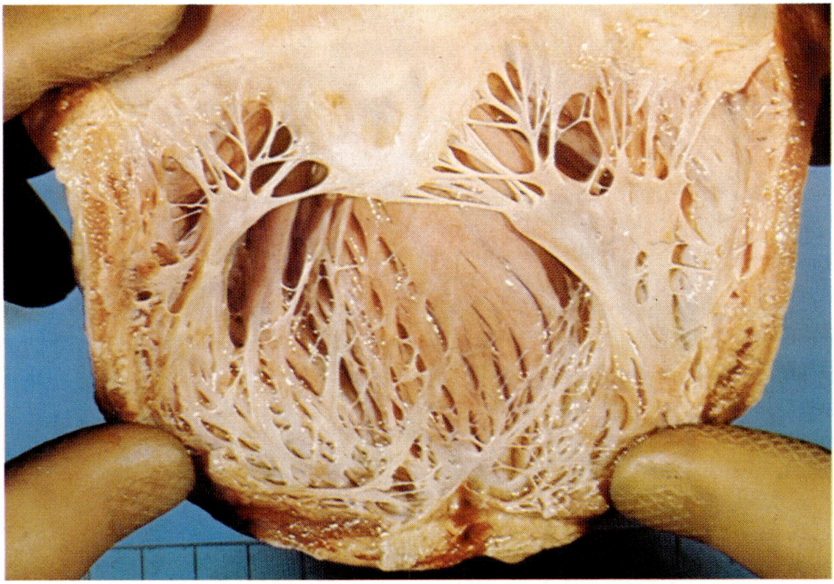

Polyarteritis nodosa

Of all the connective tissue disorders, this in particular has been looked upon as a hypersensitivity disease. The initial symptoms are so diverse that diagnosis is usually difficult. Unexplained fever, hypertension, muscle and joint pains, asthma, peripheral neuropathies, or acute abdominal pain may each be the presenting feature. Renal involvement is a later phenomenon.

The basic pathology involves the small and medium sized arteries with inflammatory changes in the media, later involving both the intima and adventitia. Destruction of the internal elastic lamina may follow, giving rise to thrombosis, or weakening of the arterial wall and aneurysm formation.

Possible related forms of primary arterial disease include cranial arteritis, Takayasu's disease (aortic arch syndrome), and Wegener's granulomatosis.

195 Typical changes of inflammation of all coats of the vessel. Note destruction of the internal elastic lamina and proliferation of the intima. This often proceeds to thrombosis in the vessel. (× *100*)

196 Focal glomerulonephritis with marked distortion of the structure of the tuft. As in the previous two diseases, renal involvement is common, occurring in over 60% of patients. Proteinuria and/or haematuria may precede hypertension and lead to renal failure.

197 A renal interlobular artery with necrosis and heavy cellular infiltration of the wall shown in another section of kidney. (× *100*)

198 Temporal arteritis (cranial arteritis). Biopsy of a temporal artery shows diffuse fibrosis of the intima with narrowing of the lumen of the vessel. The media shows inflammatory changes proceeding to focal necrosis, and giant cells may be present. This may be a benign variant of polyarteritis, occurring in an older age group. Apart from unilateral or bilateral severe temporal headache, there is often a systemic disturbance with malaise, weight loss, muscle pain and fever. (× *20*)

195

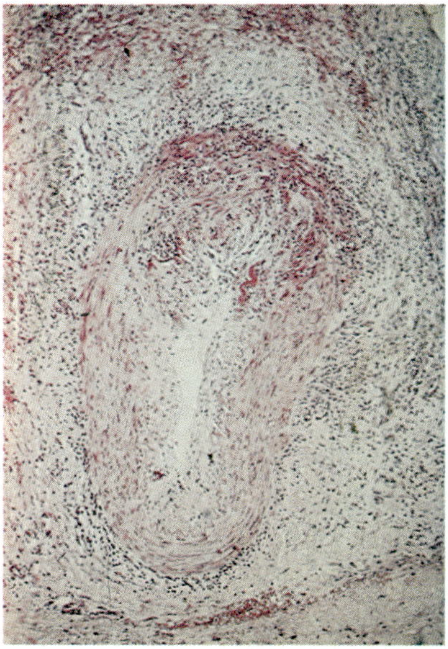

196

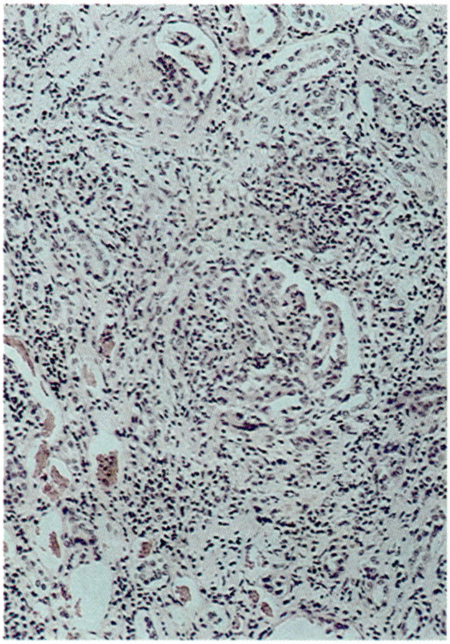

197

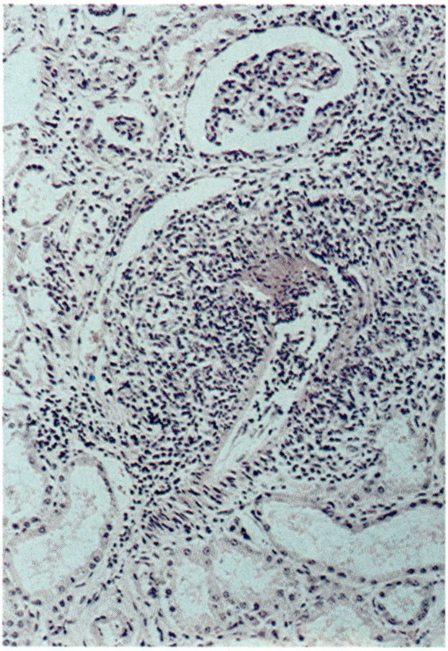

198

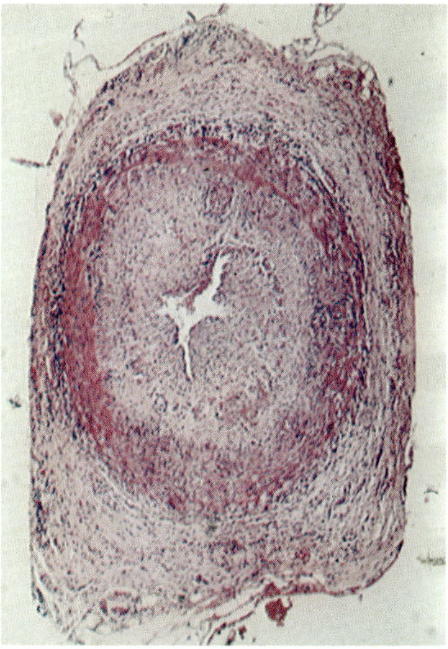

199

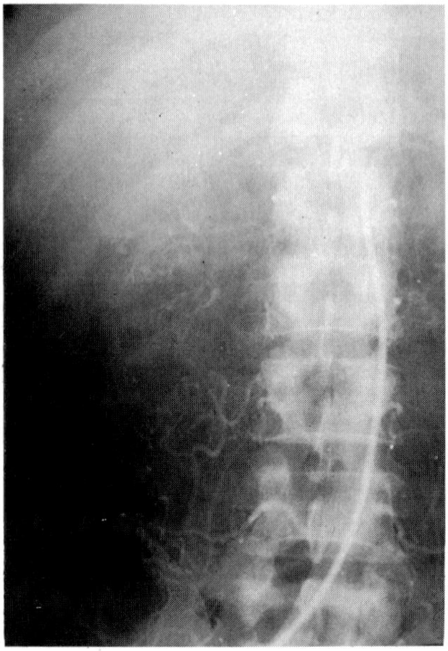

200

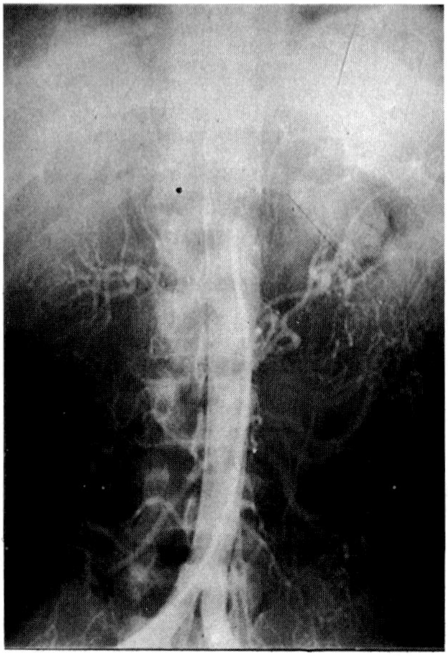

199 Aortogram in polyarteritis nodosa. Multiple microaneurysms are seen in the peripheral arterial tree.

200 Aortogram in polyarteritis nodosa, same patient (**199**).

Polymyositis

In polymyositis, the primary pathology is an inflammatory and degenerative change in skeletal muscles. The outstanding clinical feature is pain in the proximal limb segments, and examination discloses tenderness and usually profound weakness of the limbs. Polymyositis may appear as an apparently primary condition, but may also be found as part of other connective tissue disorders, especially scleroderma. Dermatomyositis is a closely related disease, in which, in addition to the findings in the muscles, an oedematous dusky red erythema occurs affecting the face and upper trunk. Both conditions, especially dermatomyositis, have a known association with malignant disease, and may precede the appearance of the latter by many months. Apart from alteration in muscle enzymes, the diagnosis may be established by muscle biopsy.

201 Typical changes of fragmented and degenerate muscle fibres lie in a background of fibrous tissue heavily infiltrated by leucocytes. (× *125*)

201

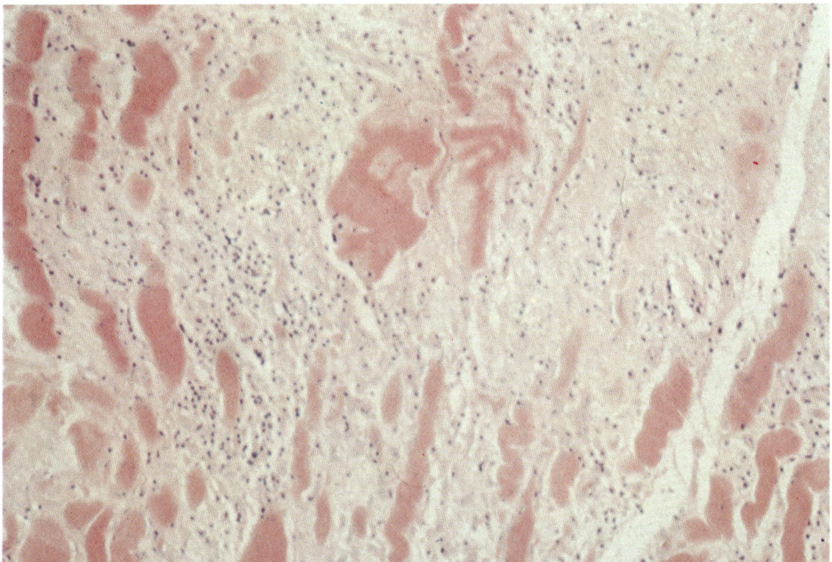

202 **Necrosis of fibres** and round cell infiltration shown in section of striated muscle. (× *125*)

203 **Hands in dermatomyositis.** Patchy erythema on the dorsum of the digits, with violaceous discoloration of the nail beds is typical.

204 **Facial eruption of dermatomyositis.** The rash is a dusky erythema involving particularly the peri-orbital region and forehead, but may also occur in the neck, shoulders and arms.

205 The typical heliotrope discoloration and oedema of the peri-orbital region, shown in close-up of same patient (**204**).

202

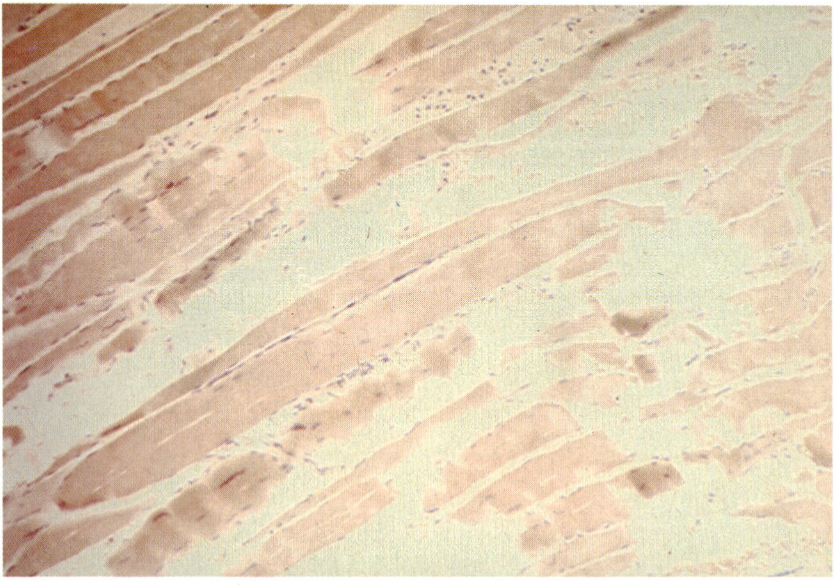

203

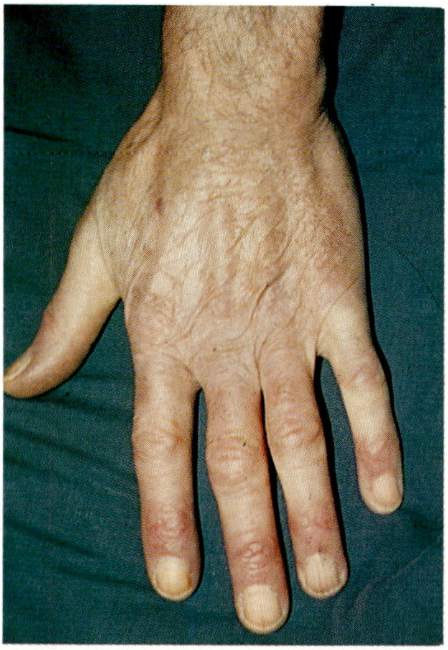

204

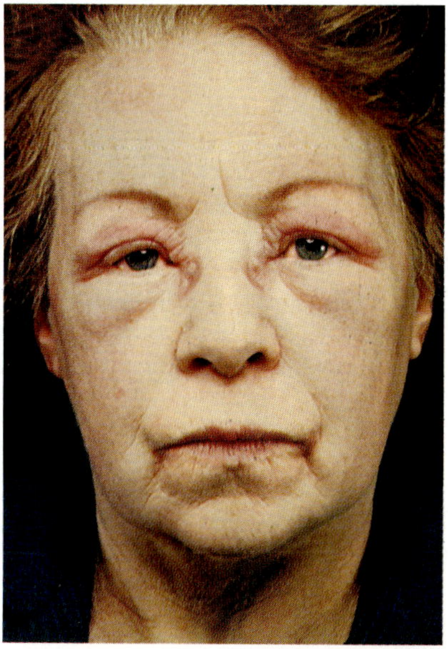

205

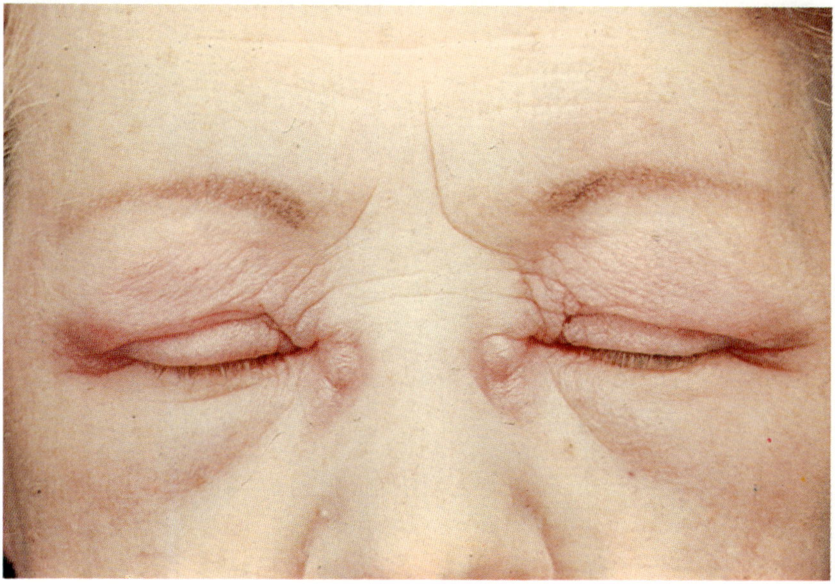

Mixed connective tissue disease

Recently recognised has been the occurrence of an 'overlap' syndrome, where the features of two or more of the connective tissue diseases appear in the same patient. Most commonly this is a mixture of the features of scleroderma and dermatomyositis, with both skin and muscle abnormalities, and often peripheral neuropathies. Some features of SLE may also occur making a definitive diagnosis difficult.

An important prognostic point is that unlike 'pure' SLE or systemic sclerosis, renal involvement is usually mild or absent.

Helpful investigations are:

(a) That on immunofluorescence a 'speckled' pattern is found on ANF testing with antibody against extractable nuclear antigen.

(b) High titres of antibody to ribonucleoprotein antigen are found.

206 Mixed connective tissue disease, immunofluorescence showing a speckled pattern of anti-nuclear antibody.

206

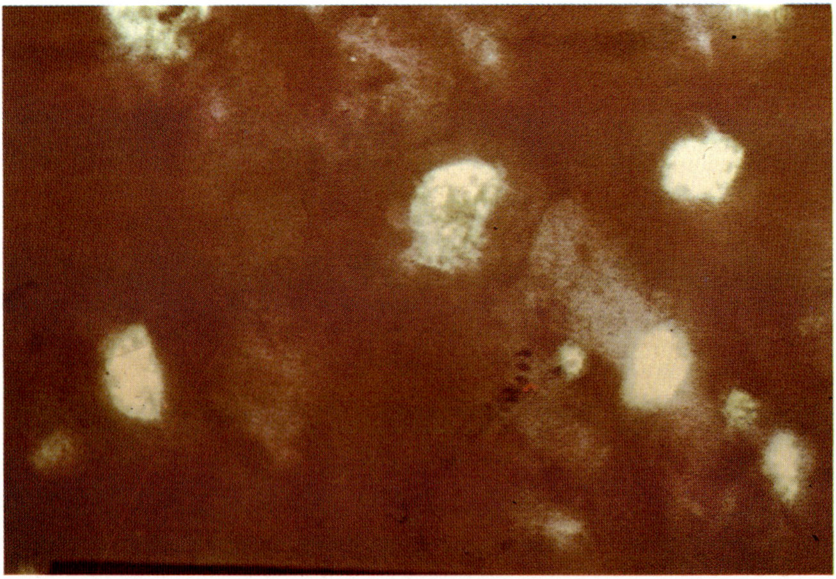

7 Rarer forms of arthritis

There are more than 100 diseases with which an arthritis may be associated, and the list on page 9 shows the more important of these. Thus an inflammatory arthritis may complicate viral infections such as rubella or glandular fever, bacterial infections as in brucellosis, gonorrhoea, or the salmonella group, hypersensitivity states, or the connective tissue disorders.

An arthritis of degenerative type may occur in endocrine disorders e.g. acromegaly, or in various metabolic diseases such as haemochromatosis. The list is large, and an underlying primary disease must always be considered if an arthritis appears in any way to vary from the common pattern.

The chapter which follows describes a few diseases in which affection of joints is by no means uncommon, and which may trap the unwary clinician.

Acromegalic arthritis

Joint pain and muscle weakness are common features of this condition. Apart from joints distended by a large effusion, acromegalic arthritis is the only form of joint disease which exhibit widening of the joint space on X-ray. Joints so affected are subject to premature and often severe degenerative changes.

207

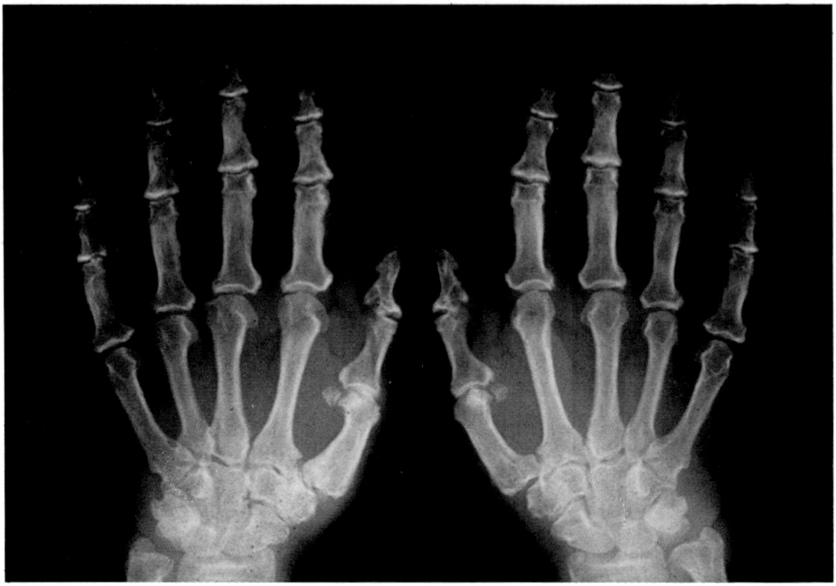

207 Large spade-like hands. There is widening of joint spaces due to hypertrophy of cartilage, tufting of terminal phalanges, and spicule osteophytes at joint margins together with ossification at muscle attachments.

208

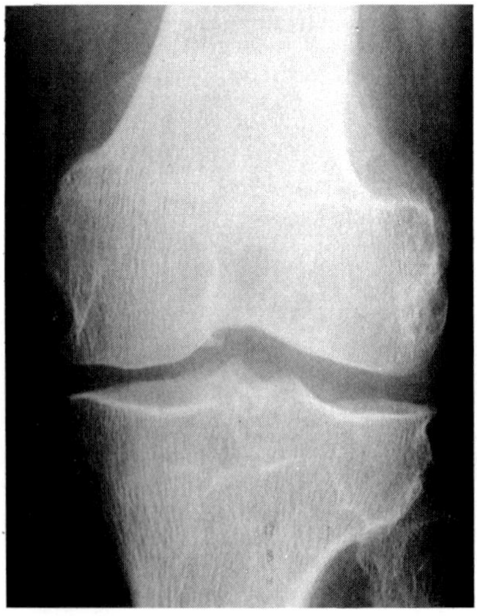

208 Acromegalic arthritis of the knee. Overgrowth of cartilage is shown by a markedly increased joint space, and there is enlargement of the femoral condyles and tibial plateau.

Hypertrophic pulmonary osteoarthropathy

Although occasionally an hereditary condition, this is usually associated with intra-thoracic disease, commonly bronchial carcinoma or cyanotic heart disease, but may also occur in chronic bowel disease.

209

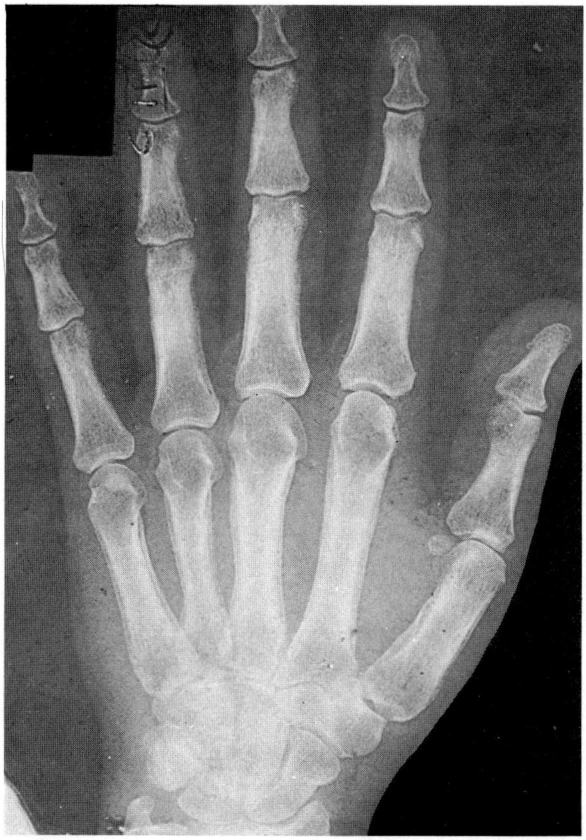

209 A fine periosteal frill along the sides of the phalanges is the characteristic appearance on X-ray. Clubbing of the finger nails proceeds to tenderness and thickening of the digits. These changes sometimes spread to involve the lower ends of the radius and ulna.

Neuropathic arthritis

Syphilis, diabetes and syringomyelia are the most common causes of neuropathic arthritis. In syphilis, the large weight bearing joints – lumbar spine, hips and knees – are most commonly affected; in diabetes, the small joints of the foot: and in syringomyelia, the joints of the upper limb. Less common causes include peroneal muscular atrophy and various peripheral neuropathies.

210 Tabes dorsalis: patient shows early changes of destruction and fragmentation affecting the lateral tibial condyle.

211 Fragmentation now affecting the tibial plateau in same patient in a more advanced stage.

212 Tabetic neuropathic arthritis of both hips. Gross destructive changes, together with massive formation of new bone in bizarre pattern around the joints.

210

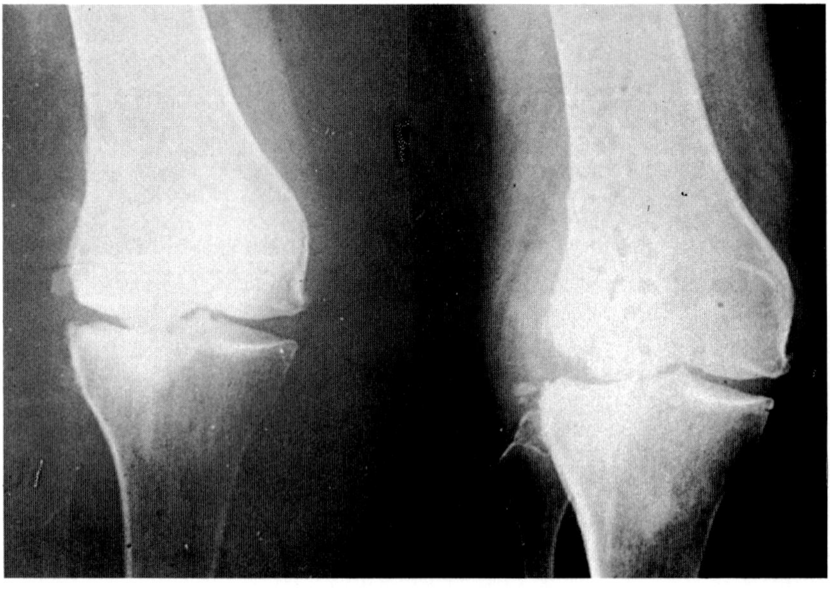

211

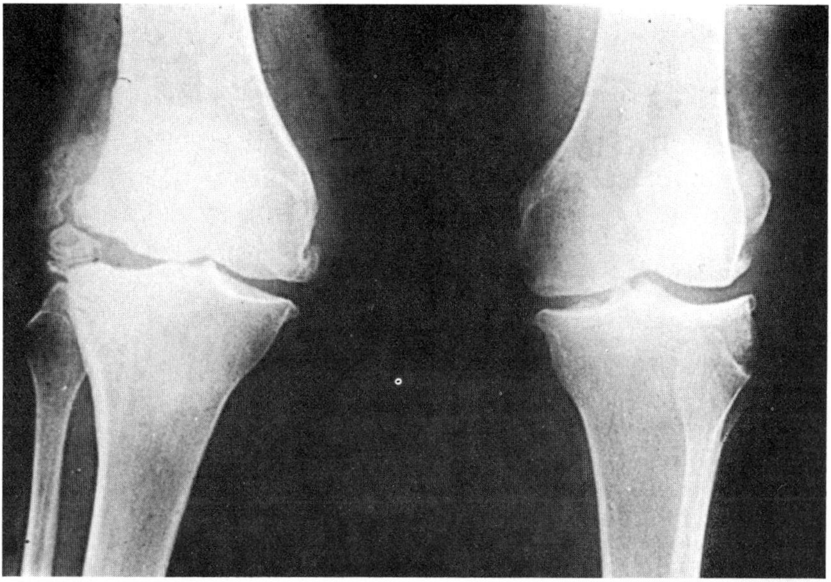

212

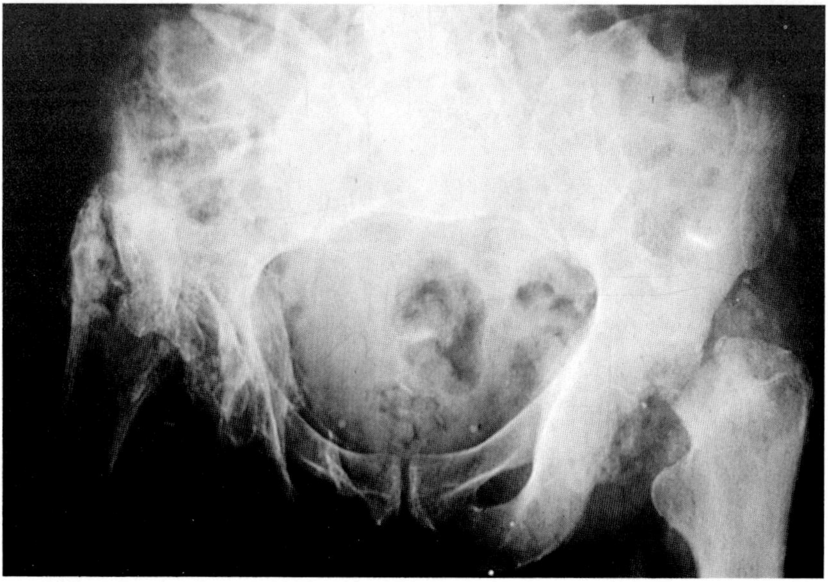

213 Neuropathic arthritis of the elbow in syringomyelia. The joint was clinically disorganised but painless on movement.

214 Destructive changes, gross new bone formation, and disorganisation of the joint are apparent in X-ray of same patient **213**.

215 Neuropathic arthritis of the ankle joint. Again destructive changes with exuberant new bone formation are seen.

216 Neuropathic arthritis of the shoulder.

213

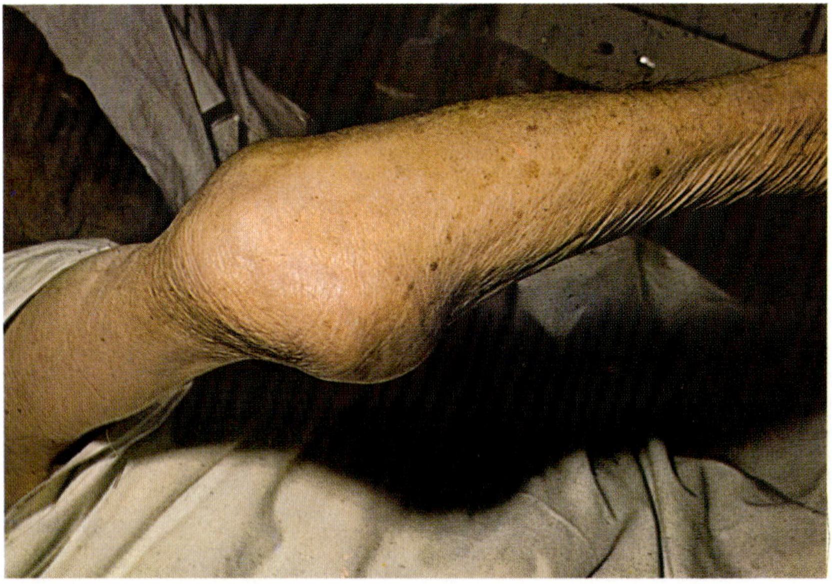

214

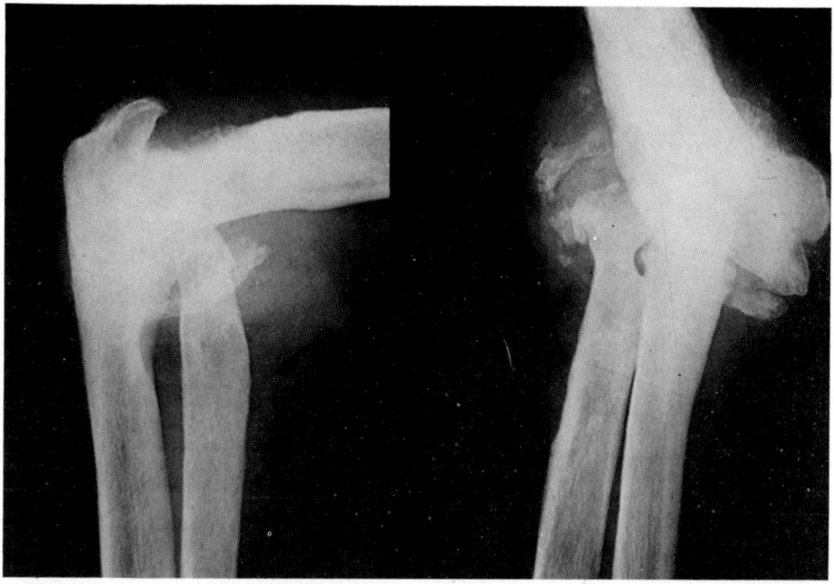

215

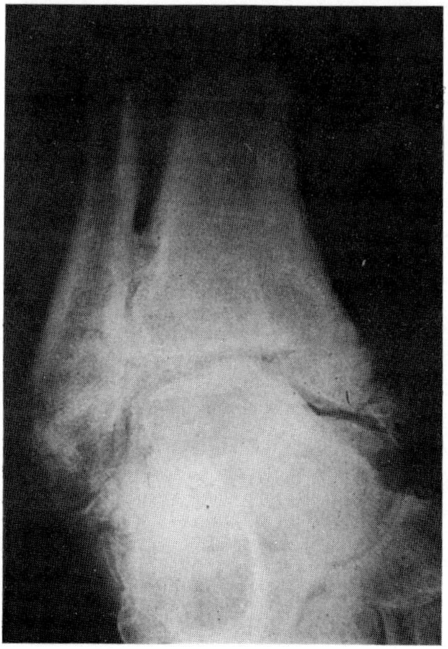

216

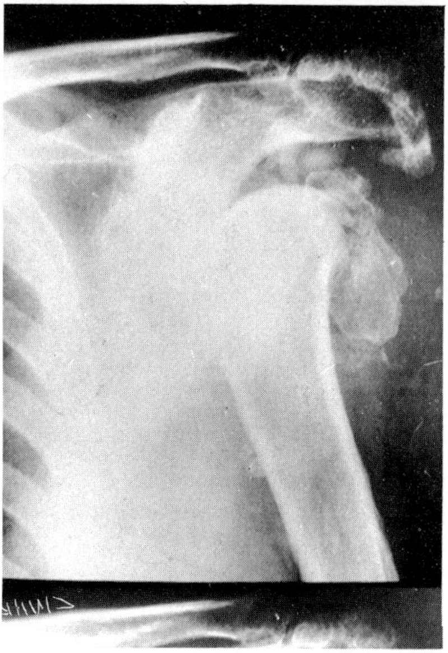

Sarcoidosis

Apart from its other manifestations such as malaise, cough, chest pain or erythema nodosum, sarcoidosis may affect muscles, bones or joints. Symptoms from muscle involvement usually amount to no more than vague aches and pains, but proximal myopathy has been described. Sarcoid of bone is usually symptomless. Arthropathy most commonly involves the knees and ankles, presenting as a symmetrical peri-arthritis or synovitis, and often precedes the onset of erythema nodosum.

217

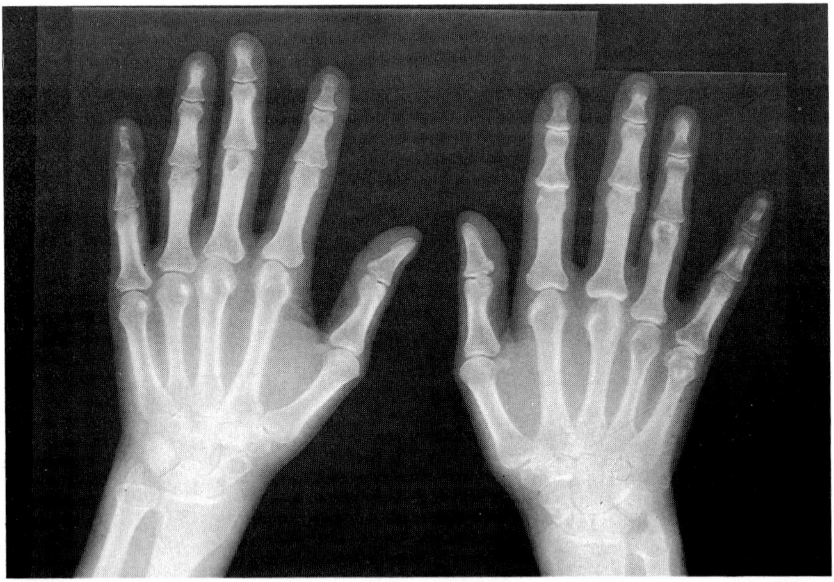

217 Central punched out areas in the phalanges are the most typical radiological change.

218 Fine lacework bone pattern in the phalanges, seen here in the middle phalanx of the ring finger, is another radiological feature in sarcoidosis.

218

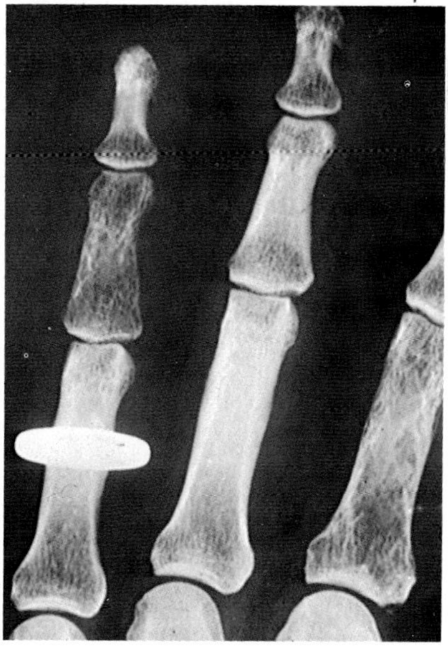

Ochronosis

This term describes the pigmentation of cartilage which occurs in those who suffer from alkaptonuria. Clinical symptoms and signs usually develop in early middle life. Bluish-black discoloration may affect the cartilage of the ears, nasal cartilage, the hard palate or the sclerae.

Joint manifestations most commonly affect the spinal column, giving the appearance of severe spondylosis. Kyphosis and ultimate rigidity of the spine results from calcification and, finally, ossification of the intervertebral discs.

Severe degenerative changes in the peripheral joints may also occur, involving the knees, hips, and shoulders.

219 Pigmentation of the nose is apparent in ochronosis.

220 Pigmentation of the sclerae shown in close-up of the same patient (**219**).

221 The ears of the same patient (**203**) display the typical bluish-black discoloration.

222 Marked collapse and calcification of intervertebral discs. Joints in ochronosis show premature and severe degenerative changes.

219

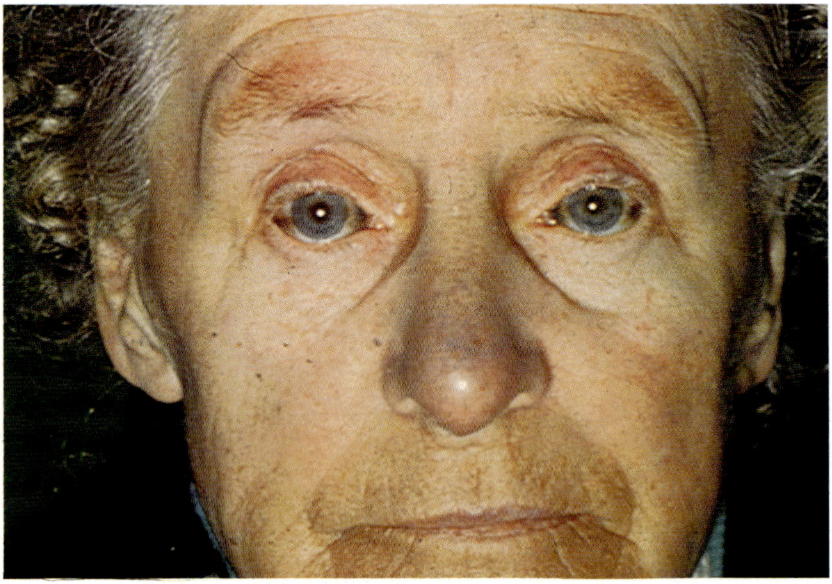

220

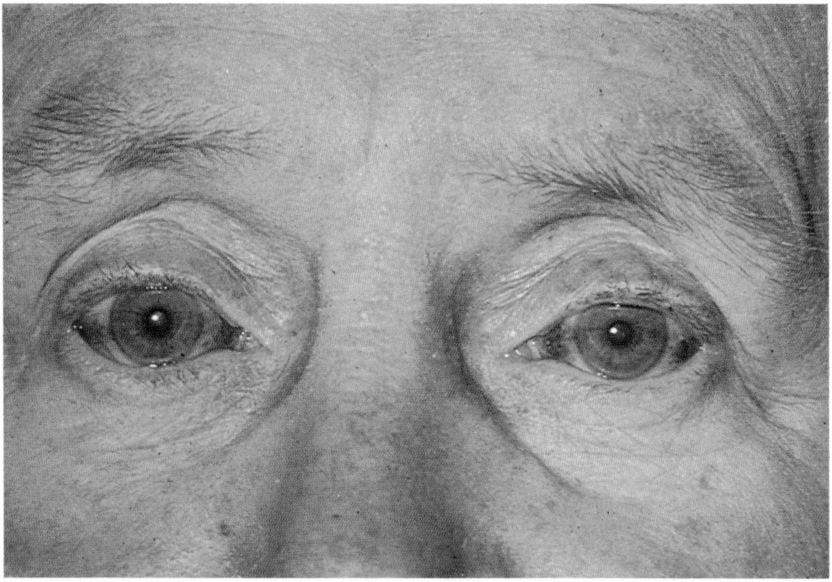

221

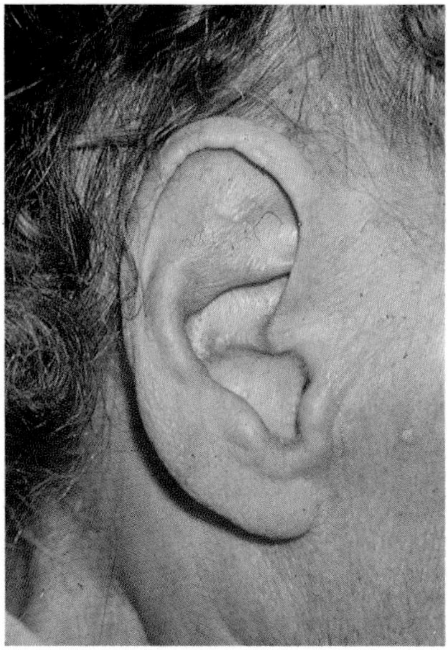

222

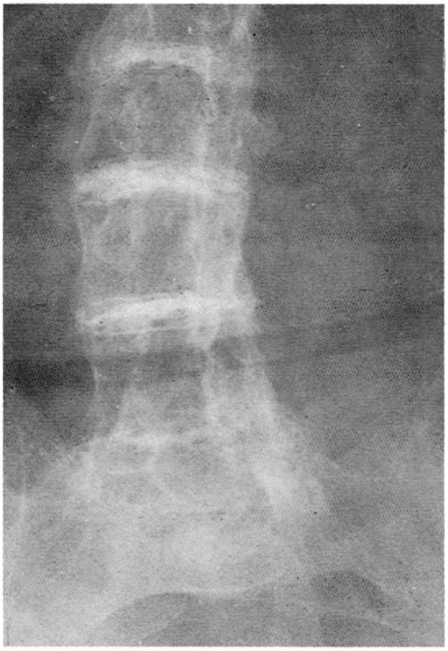

Myelomatosis

Apart from bone pain in the spine and ribs, myelomatosis is occasionally accompanied by a polyarthritis with some resemblance to rheumatoid arthritis, and involving the small joints of the hands.

223 Deposits of amyloid material cause swelling of joints. Radiologically, one may see destructive changes in bone adjacent to affected joints.

Haemochromatosis

This disease may be associated with chondrocalcinosis (see page 101), or with a more chronic and destructive arthropathy.

224 Bone sclerosis, irregularity of the joint margins and cyst formation are seen.

223

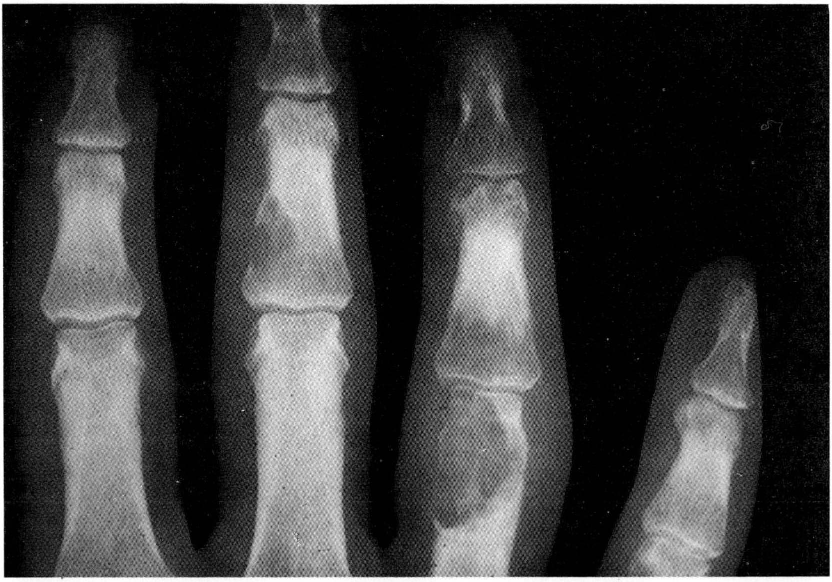

224

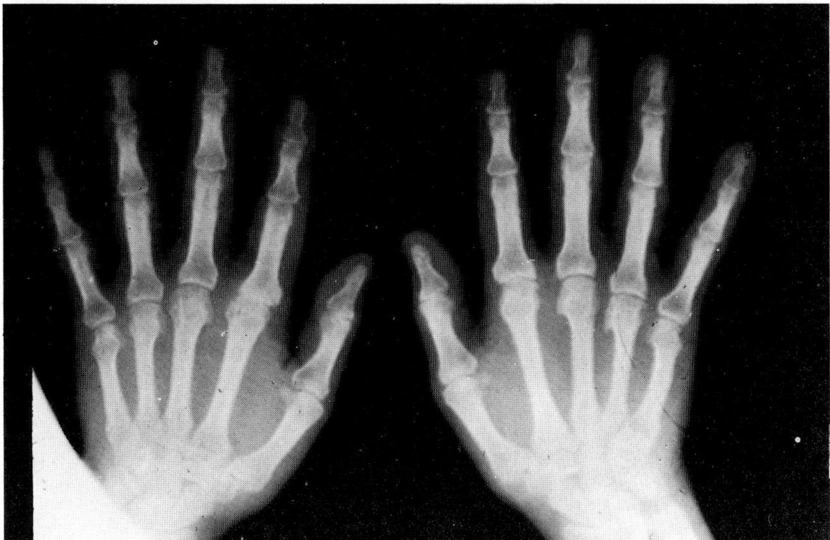

Haemophilia

The arthropathy of haemophilia is due to repeated haemarthroses. The knees, ankles, elbows, and shoulders are most commonly affected.

225 Haemophiliac knee joint. Note loss of joint space, widening of the femoral inter-condylar notch and irregular sclerotic and destructive changes affecting the tibial plateau and adjacent femoral condyle.

226 The elbow in haemophilia. Similar changes are seen as in the knee joint.

225

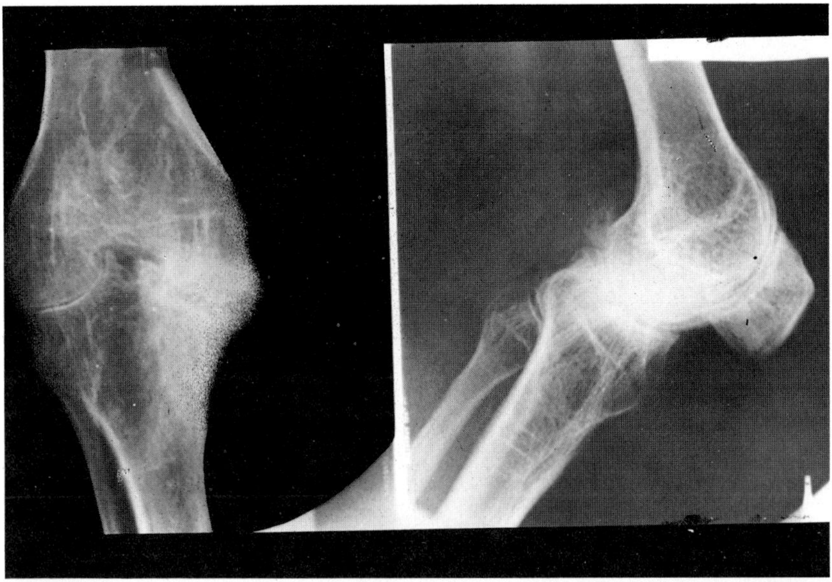

226

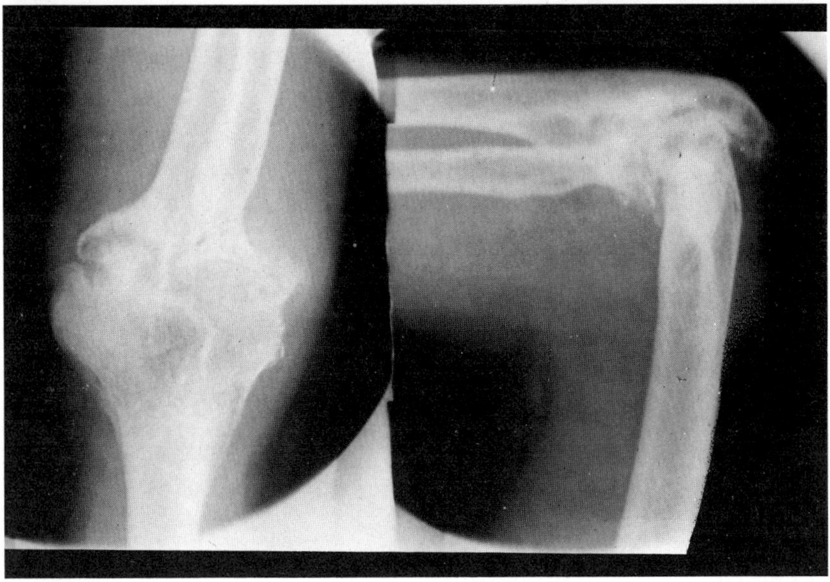

Gonococcal arthritis

Increasing resistance of the gonococcus to antibiotics has resulted in the reappearance of a septicaemic state, manifested by swollen joints and a characteristic skin rash.

227 Gonococcal arthritis of the knee presenting as a hot, swollen joint. The characteristic skin lesion is seen on the volar surface of the wrist (*arrowed*).

228 Gonococcal septicaemic skin lesions on the forearm.

227

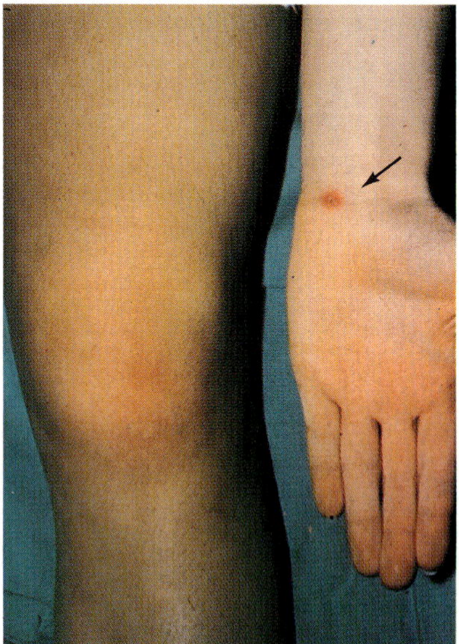

228

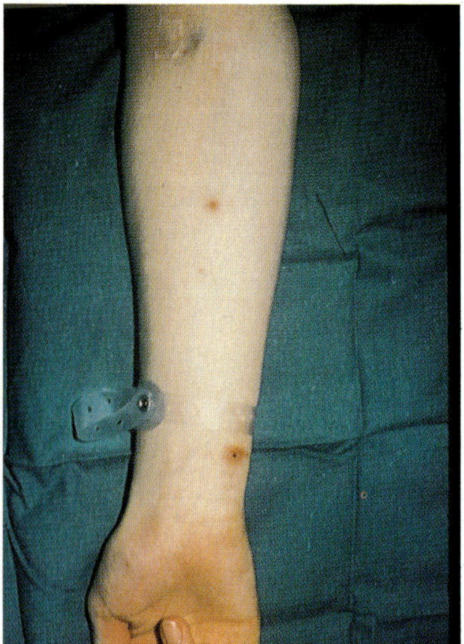

229

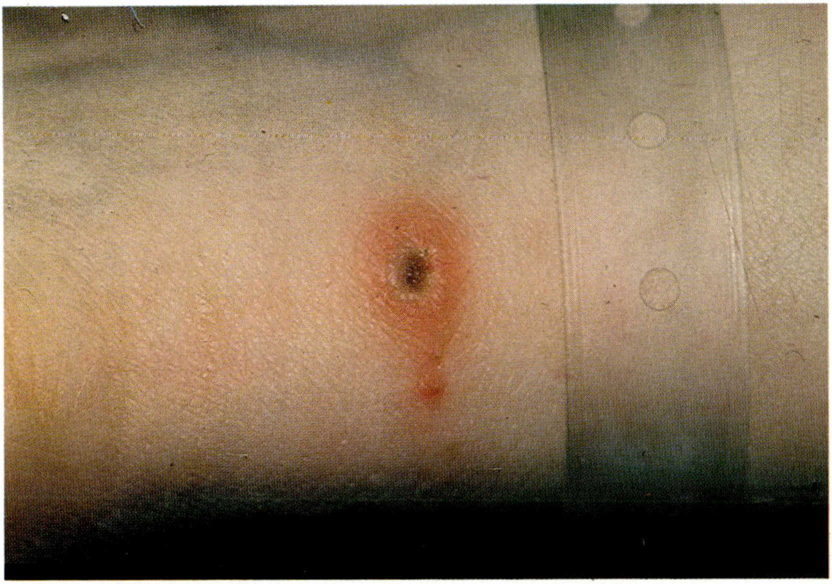

229 **Typical skin lesion:** close-up view.

Miscellaneous conditions

A wide variety of diseases, many of them not coming strictly within the province of the rheumatologist, may nevertheless have presenting symptoms of joint, muscle, or bone pain and by virtue of this will often be referred, in the first place to a rheumatological clinic.

The following illustrations show a scatter of such conditions first referred to the author's out-patient clinic.

Erythema nodosum

230

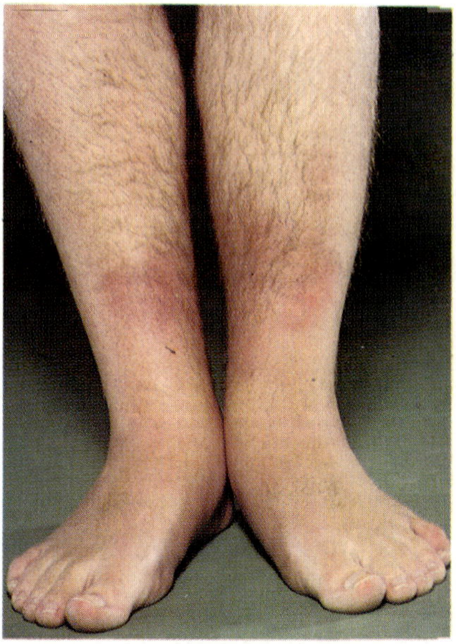

231

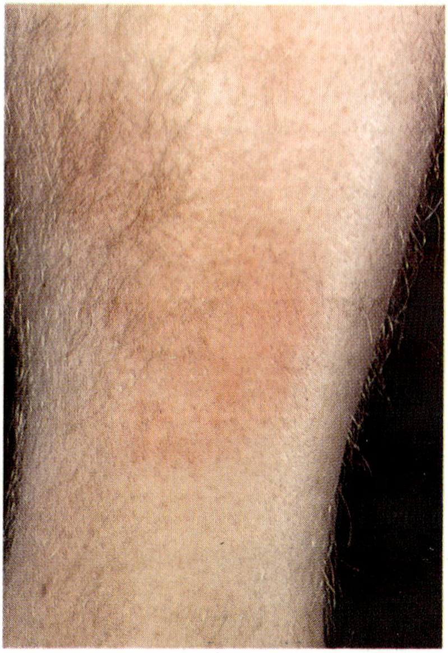

230 Typical tender raised red patches on the lower legs. Erythema nodosum is accompanied by joint manifestations in 60–75% of cases. Erythema nodosum may also occur as a manifestation of other diseases, notably streptococcal pharyngitis, rheumatic fever, tuberculosis or ulcerative colitis. It seems sometimes to occur as an idiopathic phenomenon and should be regarded as a sensitivity vasculitis.

231 Erythema nodosum: close-up view. This patient presented with a bilateral acute arthritis of the ankle joints and was found to be suffering from sarcoidosis.

Aseptic necrosis

232

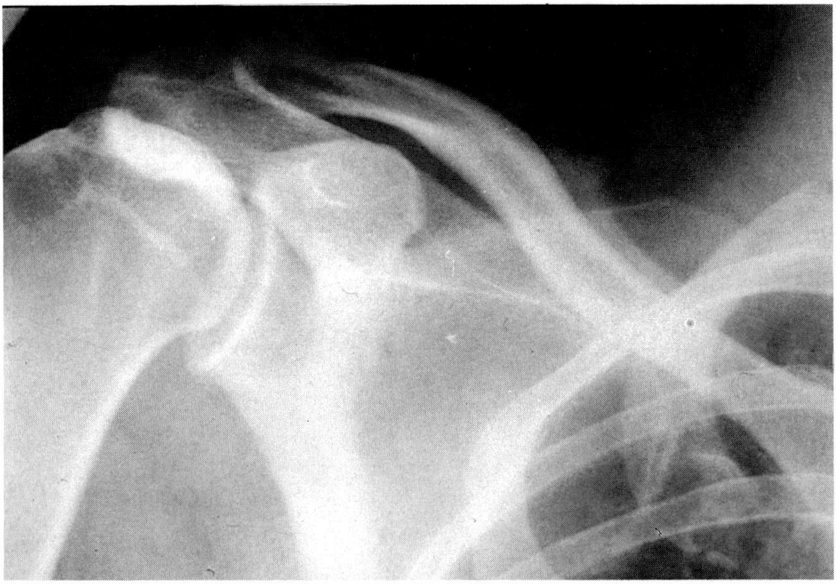

232 Aseptic necrosis of the humeral head. This and the femoral head are the common sites of this lesion. An area of dense bone is separating from the head of the humerus. Such osteonecrosis may be due to a number of systemic diseases, including sickle cell disease, Gaucher's disease, decompression sickness, alcoholism, and systemic lupus erythematosus. Longterm corticosteroid therapy has also been implicated as a cause of osteonecrosis. As would be expected, a secondary arthropathy eventually develops in joints so affected.

Gaucher's disease

This is an inherited disorder due to a specific enzyme deficiency, with widespread systemic manifestations including osteoarticular complaints due to deposition of Gaucher's cells in the long bones.

233

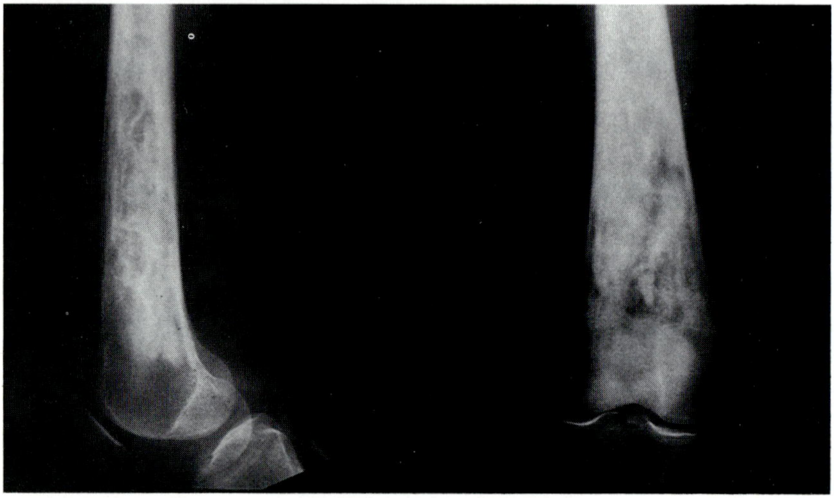

233 Typical 'Erlenmeyer flask' appearances of the lower femur showing areas of rarefaction mingled with patches of sclerosis. The patient presented complaining of pain in the knee.

234

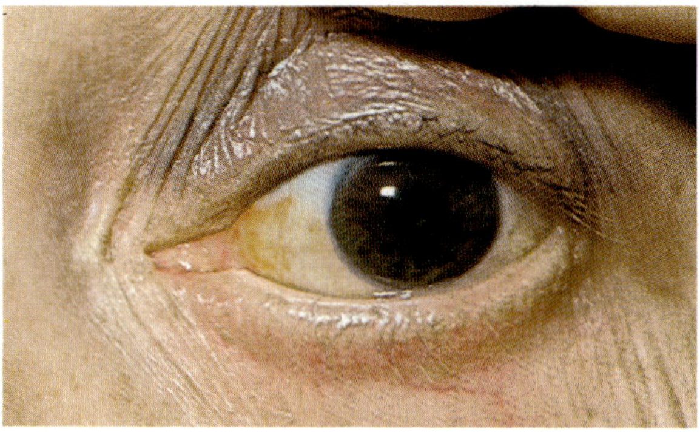

234 Gaucher's disease: the eye showing the typical pinguecula‹

Osteogenesis imperfecta

This is a heritable disorder of bone due to a defect in its acollagenous matrix. Multiple fractures may occur. The clue to diagnosis is the blue sclerae which are almost always present.

235

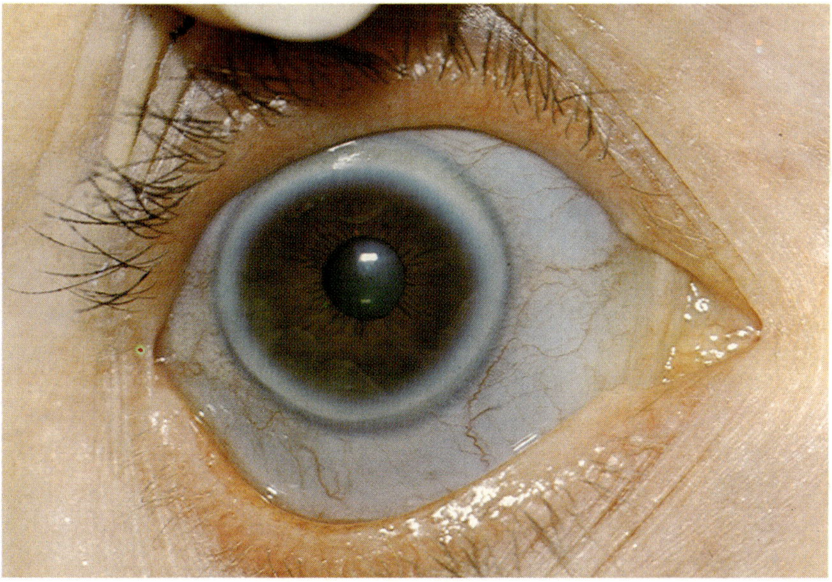

235 Typical blue sclera in osteogenesis imperfecta.

Metabolic bone disease

Rheumatic symptoms are usually the early complaint of patients suffering from the various forms of metabolic bone disease – osteomalacia and rickets due to defective supply of vitamin D, primary or secondary hyperparathyroidism, post-menopausal osteoporosis, and Paget's disease. Radiological changes may be characteristic.

236 Hyperparathyroidism: X-ray of the hands. There is marked bone resorption with mineral loss, particularly along the cortical surfaces of the proximal and distal phalanges, and gross resorption of the distal phalanges. Marked soft tissue calcification is also seen.

237 Hyperparathyroidism: X-ray of the skull showing the typical 'ground glass' appearance.

238 Hyperparathyroidism: X-ray of the knee. Apart from the changes in bone pattern, soft tissue calcification is seen, and also calcification of the menisci, indicating associated chondrocalcinosis (see page 101).

239 Post-menopausal osteoporosis: X-ray of the spine showing typical 'cod fish' appearance of the vertebral bodies, and partial collapse of the upper vertebrae.

236

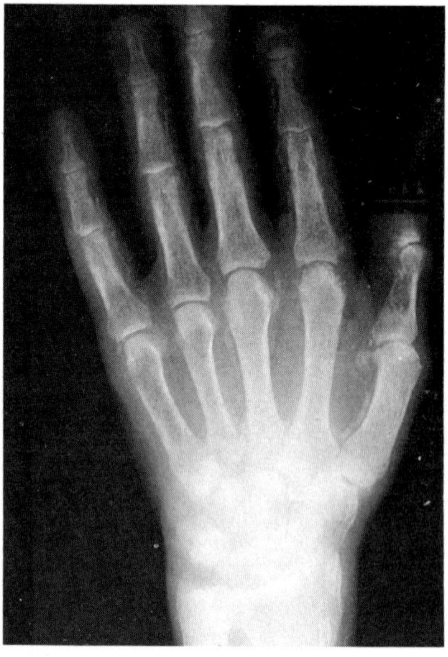

237

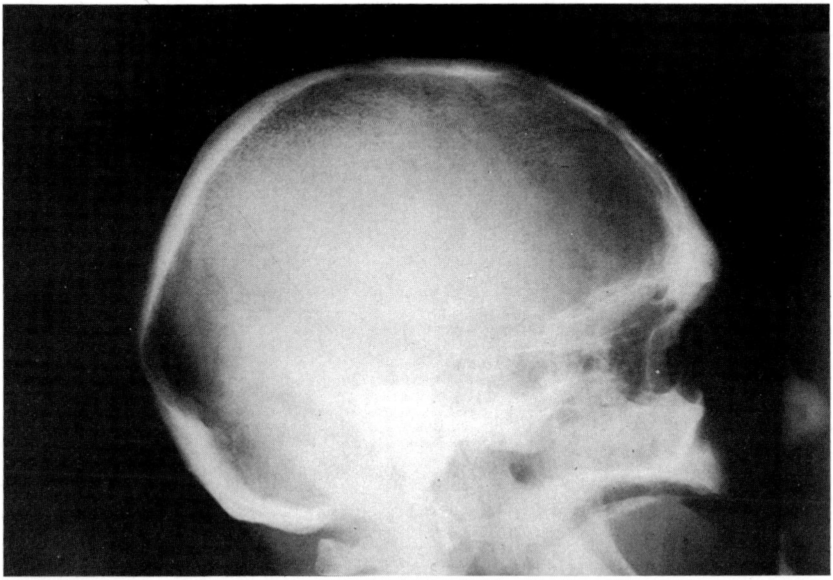

238

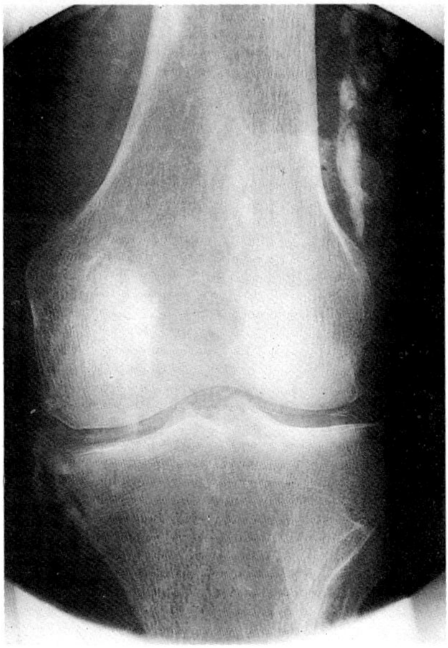

239

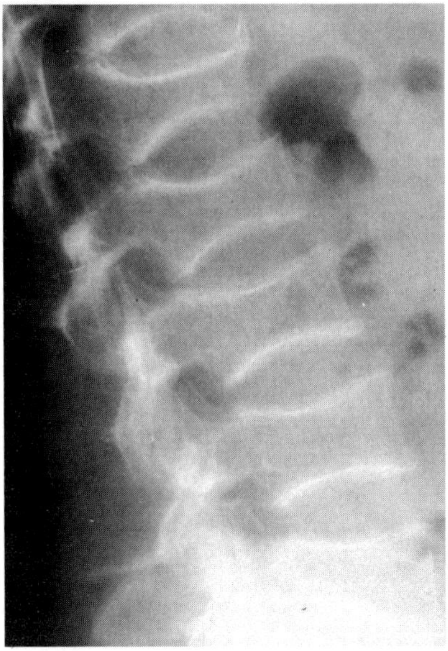

240

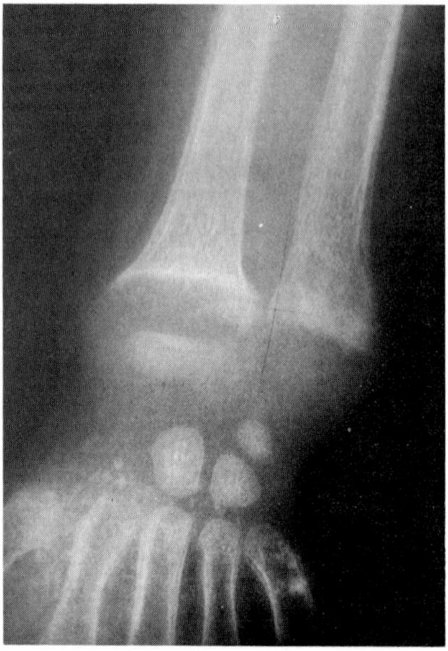

241

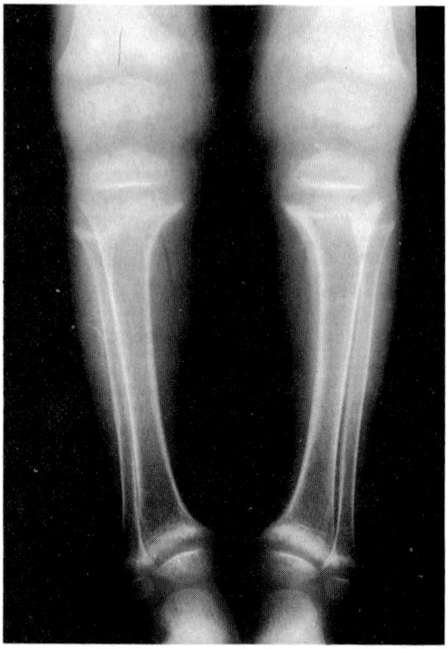

240 Child with rickets: X-ray of the wrists showing cupping of the metaphyses and enlargement of epiphyseal plates.

241 The knees of the same child (**240**) showing similar changes.

The hypermobility syndrome

Undue laxity of joints, often familial, may give rise to premature degenerative changes in later life. The cardinal signs of this condition are as illustrated in **242–246**. It probably represents an extreme of the normal variation in joint mobility, although more recent investigation into such patients suggests that thcy are unduly liable to develop chondrocalcinosis with advancing age.

242 **Hyperextension of little finger** to at least 90°.

242

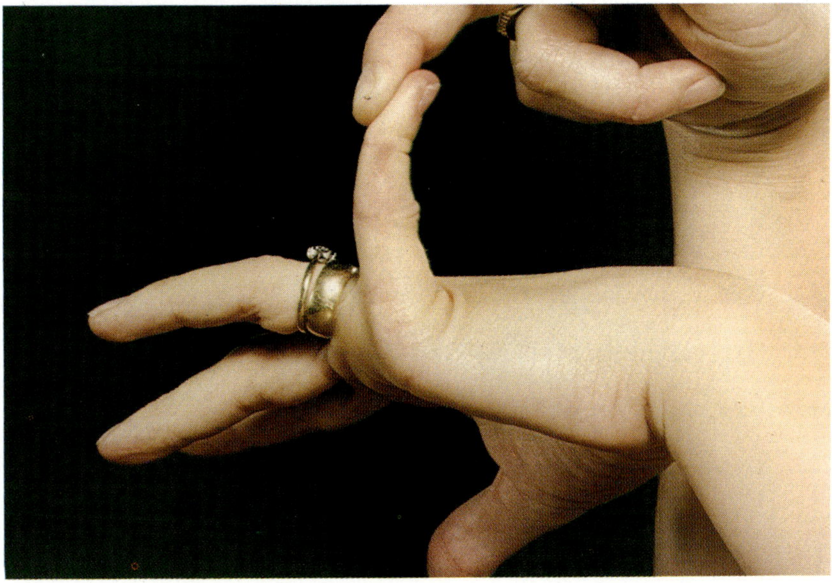

243

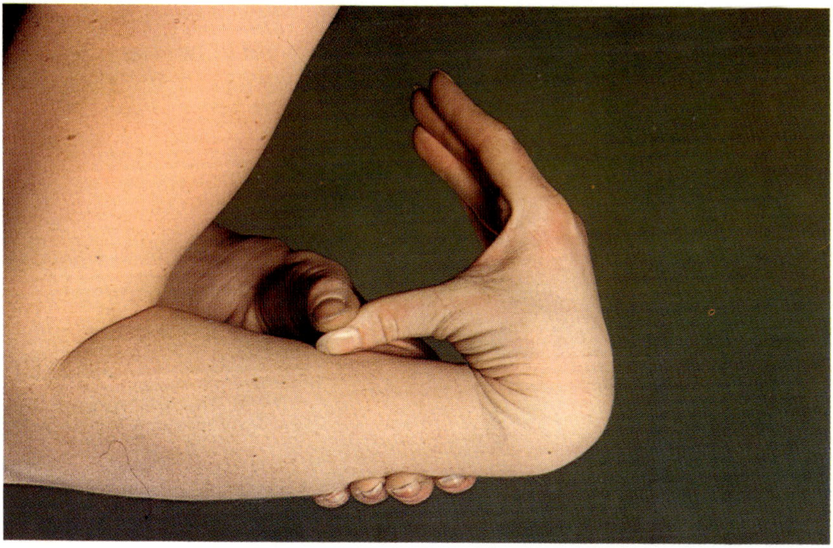

244

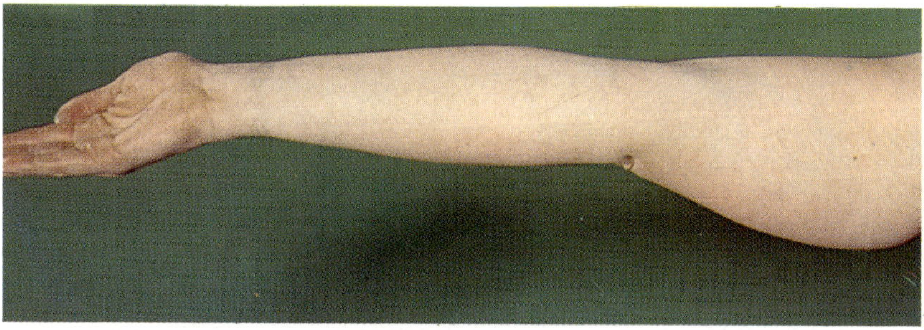

243 **Hyperextension of wrist** enabling the thumb to touch the forearm.

244 **Hyperextension of elbows** (and of the knees) is another feature.

245 **Hyperflexion of the lumbar spine and hips.**

246 **Hyperextension of the knees** (genu recurvatum).

245

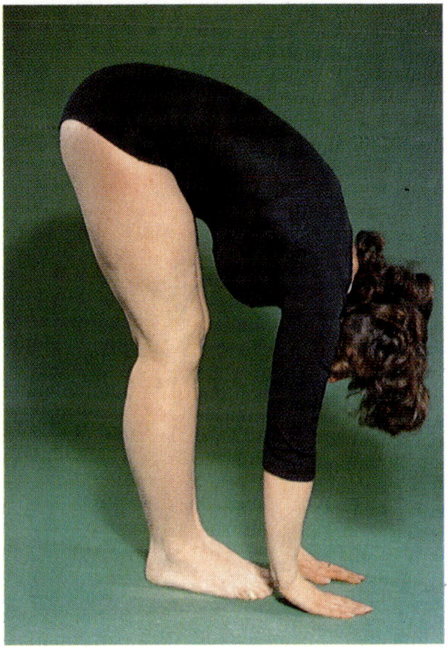

246

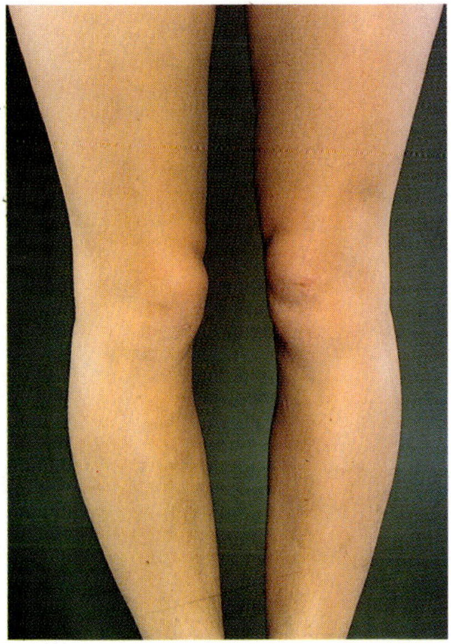

Thyroid disease

247

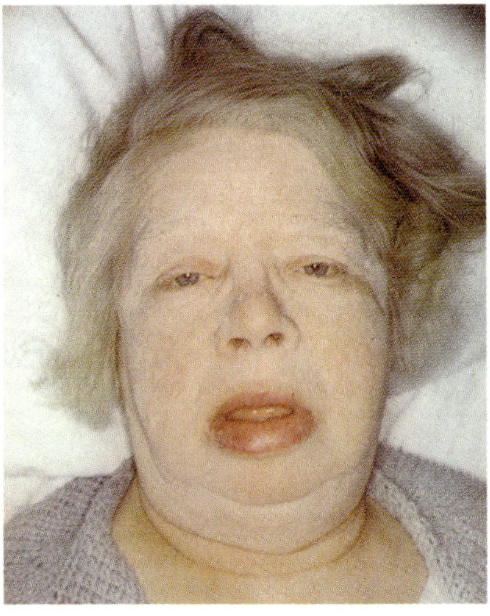

247 Myxoedema, not always clinically obvious, may first present as generalised aches and pains in muscles and joints.

248

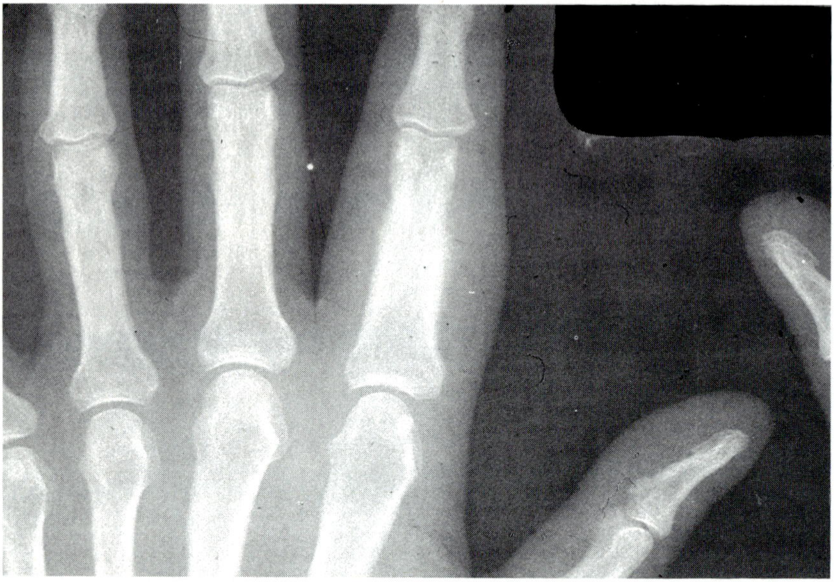

249

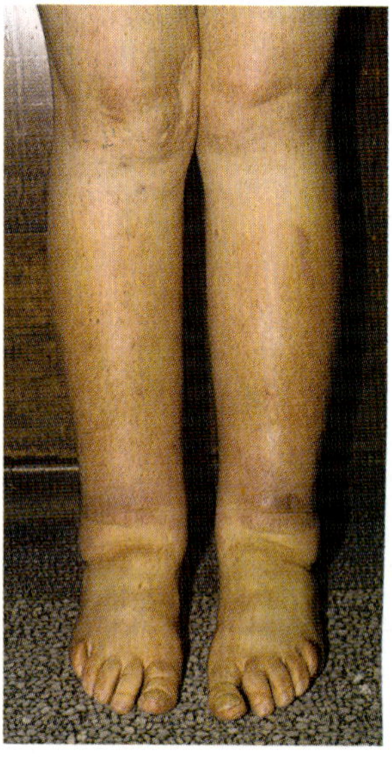

248 Thyroid acropachy. Fluffy periosteal new bone formation along the shafts of the phalanges with overlying soft tissue swelling which may be mistaken for an inflammatory arthritis.

249 Pre-tibial myxoedema often accompanies thyroid acropachy. The skin is shiny and has an 'orange peel' appearance.

250

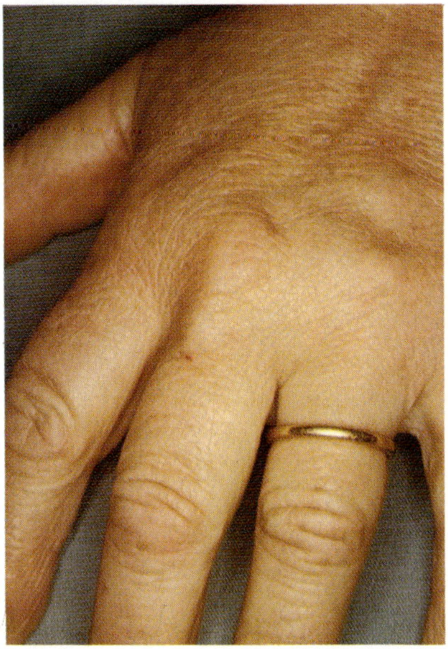

251

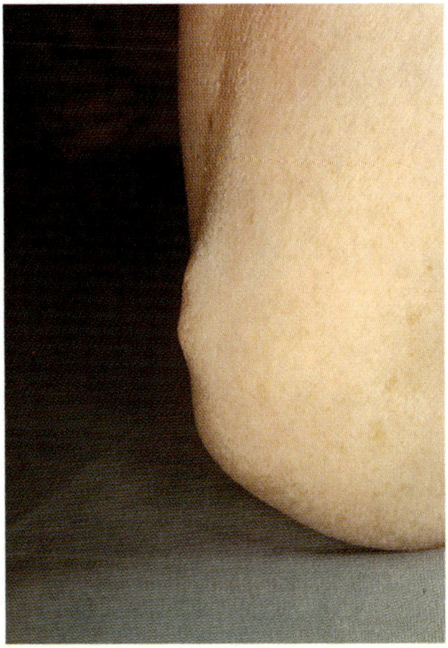

250 Some of the hyperlipoproteinaemias may present with nodules around joints resembling those seen in rheumatoid arthritis. This patient had xanthomatous deposits in the extensor tendon sheath of the middle finger.

251 Xanthomatous deposit on the elbow resembling a rheumatoid nodule.

Pigmented villo-nodular synovitis

252

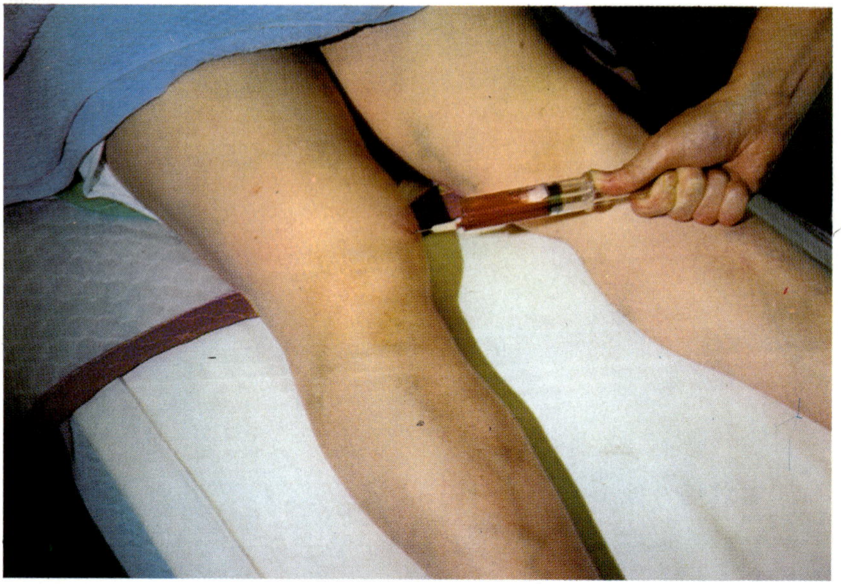

252 Inflammatory granuloma. This unusual condition commonly affects the knee joint, the patient presenting with persistent pain and swelling. Its nature is unknown, but appears basically to be an inflammatory granuloma. It should be suspected if aspiration of joint fluid is heavily blood stained as shown here.

Paget's disease of bone

253 Paget's disease: X-ray of the knee. This condition of unknown aetiology is usually asymmetrical and localised. X-ray features are bony enlargement, sometimes with deformity and replacement of normal architecture by coarse trabeculation with area of both sclerosis and lysis.

254 Localised Paget's disease affecting the 12th thoracic vertebra.

255 Paget's disease affecting the left hemi-pelvis.

253

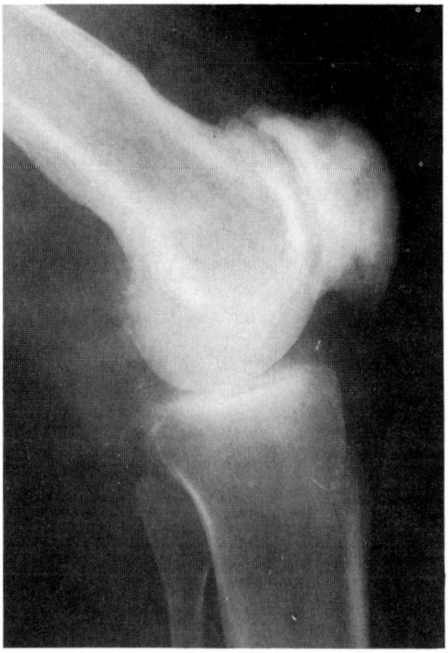

254

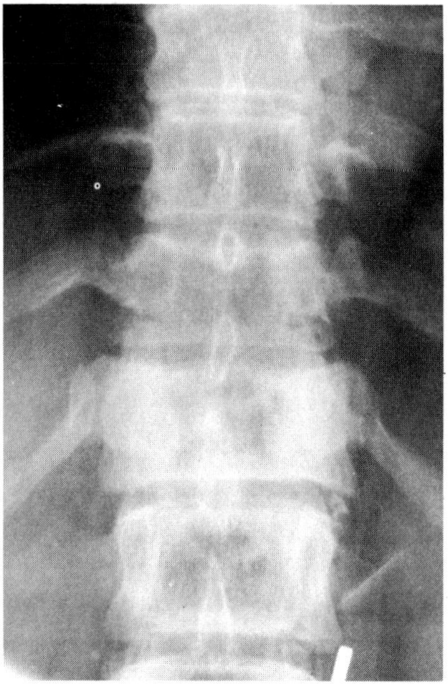

255

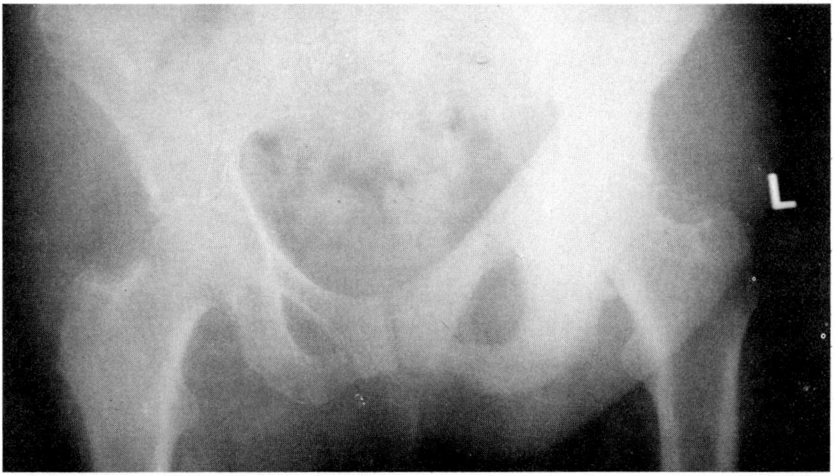

256

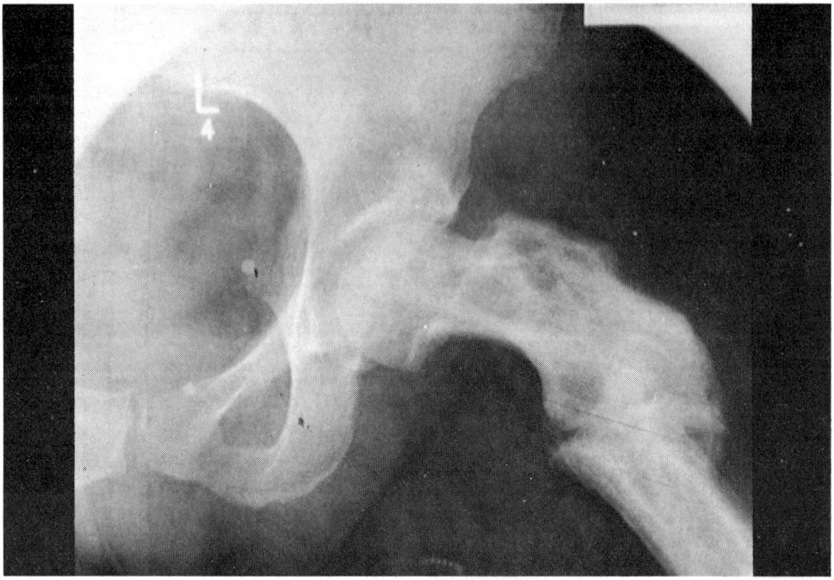

257

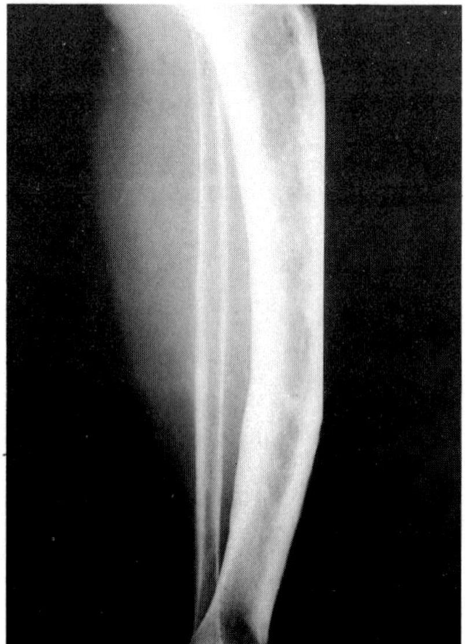

256 Pathological fractures may occur through affected bone as seen here in the upper femoral shaft.

257 Bowing of the tibia in Paget's disease.

Fluorosis

Fluoride is a natural constituent of sea water and many fresh water supplies and is important in optional concentrations for stabilising the structure of teeth and bones.

258 Osteosclerosis, trabecular coarsening and peri-osteal new bone formation: shown in X-ray of the lumbar spine. This is an intoxication of bone due to either drinking water with a high fluoride content, or accidental ingestion of fluoride-containing insecticides. Secondary degenerative joint disease commonly follows.

258

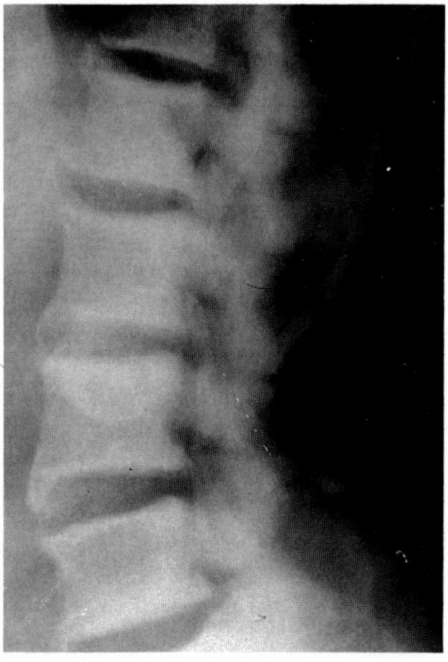

259

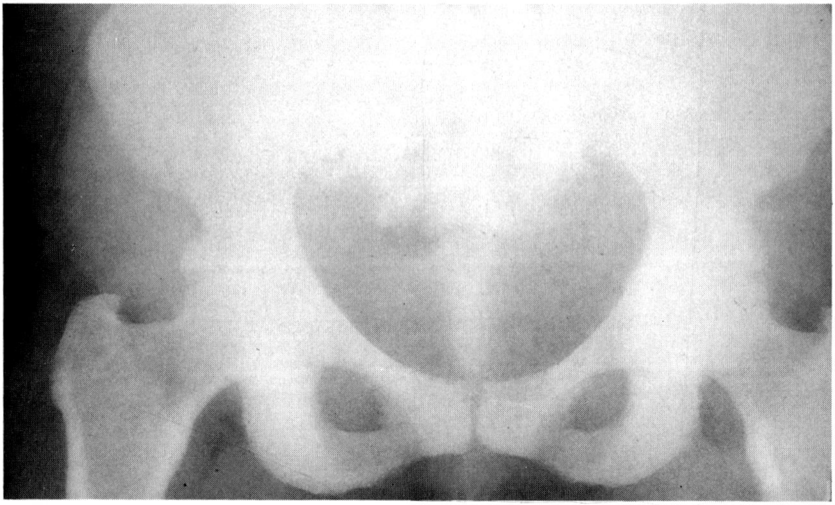

259 **The pelvis in fluorosis** showing dense osteosclerosis.

260

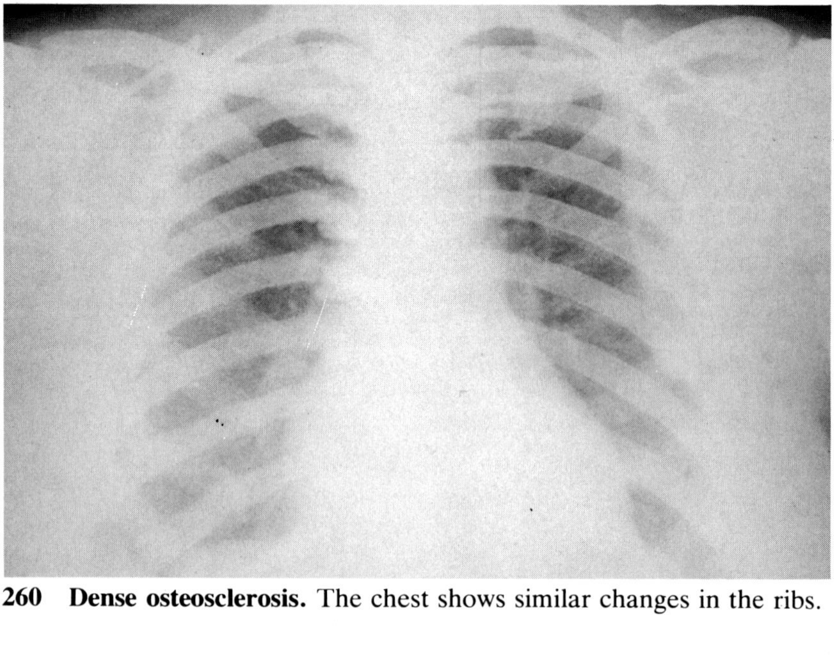

260 **Dense osteosclerosis.** The chest shows similar changes in the ribs.

Index

(The references printed in **bold** type refer to picture and caption numbers, those in light type refer to page numbers.)